Lecture Notes on Paediatrics

To medical secretaries everywhere,
and especially to those who
have helped us to prepare six editio
of this book over 18 years

Lecture Notes on Paediatrics

S.R. MEADOW
MA, BM, FRCP, DCH, DRCOG
*Professor of Paediatrics and
Child Health (St. James's)
University of Leeds
Honorary Consultant Paediatrician*

R.W. SMITHELLS
MD, FRCP, FRCP(E), DCH
*Emeritus Professor of Paediatrics and
Child Health (Leeds General Infirmary)
University of Leeds*

SIXTH EDITION

FOUR DRAGONS

LONDON EDINBURGH BOSTON

MELBOURNE PARIS BERLIN VIENNA

© 1973, 1975, 1978, 1981, 1986, 1991 by
Blackwell Scientific Publications
Editorial Offices:
Osney Mead, Oxford OX2 0EL
25 John Street, London WC1N 2BL
23 Ainslie Place, Edinburgh EH3 6AJ
3 Cambridge Center, Cambridge,
 Massachusetts 02142, USA
54 University Street, Carlton
 Victoria 3053, Australia

Other Editorial Offices:
Arnette SA
2 rue Casimir-Delavigne,
75006 Paris,
France

Blackwell Wissenschaft
Meinekestrasse 4,
D-1000 Berlin 15,
Germany

Blackwell MZV
Feldgasse 13,
A-1238 Wien,
Austria

First published 1973
Revised reprint 1974
Second edition 1975
Reprinted 1977
Third edition 1978
Reprinted 1981
Fourth edition 1981
Reprinted 1985
Fifth edition 1986
Reprinted 1990
Sixth edition 1991
Four Dragons edition 1991

Portuguese translation 1980
Asian edition 1983

Set by Semantic Graphics, Singapore
Printed and bound in Great Britain
by Hartnolls Ltd, Bodmin, Cornwall

DISTRIBUTORS

Marston Book Services Ltd
PO Box 87,
Oxford OX2 0DT
(Orders: Tel: 0865 791155
           Fax: 0865 791927
           Telex: 837515)

USA
 Mosby-Year Book, Inc.
 11830 Westline Industrial Drive,
 St Louis, Missouri 63146
 (Orders: Tel: 800 633-6699)

Canada
 Mosby-Year Book, Inc.
 5240 Finch Avenue East,
 Scarborough, Ontario
 (Orders: Tel: 416 298-1588)

Australia
 Blackwell Scientific Publications
  (Australia) Pty Ltd
 54 University Street,
 Carlton, Victoria 3053
 (Orders: Tel: 03 347-0300)

British Library
Cataloguing in Publication Data

Meadow, Roy
 Lecture notes on paediatrics.
 1. Paediatrics
 I. Title II. Smithells, R.W.
 (Richard Worthington)
 618.92

ISBN 0-632-03113-1 (BSP)
ISBN 0-632-3249-9 (Four Dragons)

Contents

Colour plates 1–7 appear between pages 182 and 183

Preface to Sixth Edition

As the 21st century approaches we are pleased to detect a growing realization that children are important. They represent the only future for mankind, the only investment with lasting dividends, the only custodians of the ideals which successive civilizations have striven to achieve. Their health, their education and —above all—their homes form the tripod upon which their future is based. We must take a lot of trouble to get them right.

World-wide, child health is affected principally by parenting, politics and public health. It is only after the basic necessities of good food, clean water, sanitation and immunization are in place that doctors make an impact on child mortality and morbidity.

Our book is designed for student doctors and other health workers in the more favoured parts of the world. We hope they will recognize their good fortune and seek ways to help children who still lack the bare essentials.

This sixth edition has been substantially revised to take account of developments and advances in recent years. It saddens us that we have had to add more about child abuse than about any other topic; nevertheless paediatrics and child health remain essentially happy and hopeful disciplines, and children the most rewarding patients to treat.

Roy Meadow
Dick Smithells
Leeds, 1991

Preface to First Edition

Paediatrics concerns the health and illness of children. Children make up more than one-fifth of our population and an even higher proportion of a general practitioner's working day. It is often in childhood that the patterns of adult health and disease have their origins. Paediatrics rubs shoulders with education and with the social services. It is concerned with children and their families first and with disease second.

Medical education is a continuing process which starts at school and should not end before retirement. The pre-registration year ensures that the new medical student is not 'let loose upon the public'. Today's medical students should therefore be expected to absorb less factual material than did their ancestors. This is a small book, intended to live in the pocket of a white coat rather than on a bookshelf. It describes the pattern of childhood growth and development and conditions that are either common, important or interesting. This factual framework is set against the changing pattern of paediatric practice, the services available for children and the needs of society.

Our aim has been to provide a framework of paediatric knowledge sufficient for the medical student during the paediatric appointment; but it must be grafted on to preliminary experience of adult medicine and surgery. We have deliberately placed more emphasis on diagnosis than on treatment; therapeutic details are best learned by caring for sick children.

For medical students who use this book, far more important than further reading is the need to spend time and trouble getting to know children, and developing the techniques of examining children and talking to them and their parents. This applies also to the many other groups who work with children—therapists, nurses and health visitors—for whom we hope this book will provide a useful supplement to their lectures and their work.

Roy Meadow
Dick Smithell

Acknowledgements

We thank our colleagues for their advice and help, and in particular Dr C.C. Bailey, Dr J.M.H. Buckler, Dr N. Cavanagh, Dr J.H.C. Evans, Dr J.M. Littlewood, Dr E.J. Simmonds and Dr J. Verbov.

The figures were drawn and most of the photographs were prepared by the Departments of Medical Illustration and Photography at the University of Leeds, and St James's University Hospital.

We are grateful to a number of colleagues who have helped with illustrations, particularly Dr P.R.F. Dear, Dr J.M. Littlewood, Professor V. Dubowitz, Professor M.I. Levene and Professor J.M. Tanner.

We are indebted to our assistant Mandy Jones for her efficient and intelligent work with the manuscripts.

Acknowledgements

We thank our colleagues for their advice and help, and in particular Dr C.C. Bailey, Dr J.M.H. Buckler, Dr N.K. Cavanagh, TX, J.H.C. Evans, Dr M.F. Eastwood, Dr E.L. Simmonds and Dr J. Verbov.

The figures were drawn and most of the photographs were prepared by the Department of Medical Illustration and Photography at the University of Leeds and St James's University Hospital.

We are grateful to a number of colleagues who have helped with illustration, particularly Dr P.F.P. Dear, Dr J.M. Littlewood, Professor V. Dubowitz, Professor M.I. Levene and Professor J.M. Tanner.

We are indebted to our assistant Mandy Jones for her efficient and intelligent work with the manuscripts.

Chapter 1
Children and their Health

Children under the age of 15 comprise 20% of the population of the UK and of most industrialized countries; but in many developing countries children represent more than 50% of the population. In all countries children provide a high proportion of a doctor's work, and in Britain many general practitioners find that 30% or more of their consultations are for children, particularly pre-school children (under 5 years). (Medical students in the middle of a 2- or 3-month paediatric attachment may wonder why only 5% of their training should be devoted to children!)

MORTALITY AND MORBIDITY

The health of nations has traditionally been measured by mortality. It seems paradoxical, but it is administratively easier to record deaths and their causes than morbidity, which is more difficult to determine, even for the few diseases (mostly infections) which are notifiable by law. Special studies are needed to determine the incidence of other conditions.

The causes of death and the patterns of illness in children differ markedly from those in adults. They are influenced by a diversity of factors which include sex, legitimacy, social class, place of birth and season of the year. The secular decline in child mortality during the present century has resulted more from preventive (public health) measures than from improved treatment. Today virtually the entire population of the UK has safe food and water, free immunization and easy access to local health care. Such is not the case for a family in a non-industrialized country.

Child mortality is concentrated in the perinatal period, and the only remaining scope for a *major* reduction in child deaths in Britain lies in better obstetric, neonatal and infant care.

Important mortality indices include:

Stillbirth rate = Stillbirths per 1000 total births
Perinatal mortality rate = Stillbirths + first week deaths per 1000 total births
Neonatal mortality rate = Deaths in first 28 days per 1000 live births
Infant mortality rate = Deaths in first year per 1000 live births

A stillbirth refers to a child born dead after the 28th week of pregnancy. A child or fetus born dead earlier in pregnancy is an abortion or miscarriage. A baby that shows signs of life (e.g. heart beat) at birth is a live birth irrespective of the length of gestation.

The national rates hide considerable regional differences: thus, although the 1988 national perinatal mortality rate was 8.7 per 1000 births, the variations in the districts of one health region (Yorkshire) were between 8 and 14 per 1000 births.

1

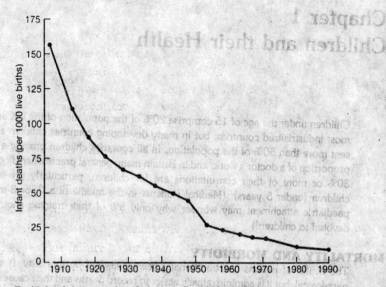

Fig. 1.1. Infant mortality (0–1 year). By 1989 the infant mortality in England and Wales had fallen to a fraction of the level in 1900 (from 156 per 1000 live births to 9 per 1000). The present rate is amongst the lowest in the world, but by no means the lowest in Europe.

The continuing fall in infant mortality (Fig. 1.1) is commendable but it is salutary to recognize that most of the Scandinavian countries, Japan and Switzerland have consistently lower rates than the UK. On the other hand, several of the East European countries have infant mortality rates 2–3 times higher (similar to Britain 40 years ago), and some of the non-industrialized countries would need to be on a different scale altogether. The improvement in infant mortality in the UK in recent years has been attributable to the reduction in neonatal mortality; post-neonatal mortality (from 1 month to 1 year) fails to show significant improvement. Sudden Infant Death Syndrome (SIDS) comprises the largest category of death in the post-neonatal period (Table 1.1). Whilst other causes of infant death have declined substantially in the last 30 years, the number of deaths classified as SIDS has changed little.

Table 1.1. Post-neonatal (1 month–1 year) mortality rates per 100 000 live births by cause of death and social class.

		Social class		
	Total	I and II	V	Unclassifiable
Sudden infant death syndrome	140	100	245	333
Congenital anomalies	80	66	105	130
Accidental	20	10	41	96
Perinatal problems	18	14	21	30

Deaths are concentrated in early life and are higher for boys at all ages, by a factor of 1.3 in the first month of life and by 1.6 for children of school age. For a schoolchild, death is more likely to be due to an accident, particularly a road accident with the child as pedestrian or cyclist, than to any disease (Table 1.1). The decline in mortality from infectious diseases has made other serious disorders appear more common. Death from malignancy is now as common as from infection (Fig. 1.2).

The pattern of morbidity in children is very different from that of adults. Though degenerative disorders and cerebral vascular accidents are very rare in childhood new forms of chronic disease are becoming relatively more important, as formerly fatal childhood disorders become treatable but not necessarily curable. Thus children with complex congenital heart disease, malignant disease, cystic fibrosis and renal failure receive treatments that all too often leave the child handicapped, either by incomplete cure or the need to live with the difficulties and side-effects of complicated treatment. Infections are common, especially of the upper and lower respiratory, gastrointestinal and urinary tracts, as well as the acute exanthemata.

The hallmarks of childhood are growth and development which influences both the kinds and the patterns of childhood illness. Congenital malformations, genetic disease and the consequences of problems in the perinatal period (e.g. cerebral palsy) are common. Disturbances of development and behaviour, as well as anxiety about normal variants, may demand a lot of the doctor's time. As an

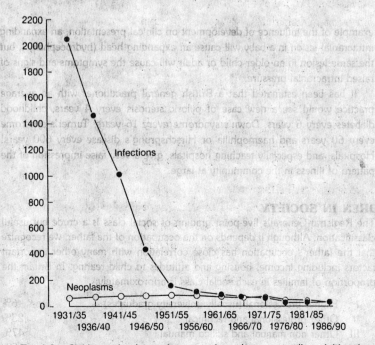

Fig. 1.2. Child mortality from infections and neoplasms, per million children living (aged 1–4 years).

Table 1.2. Episodes of childhood illness in general practice in 1 year.

	Episodes per 1000 children	
Diagnosis	0–4 years	5–14 years
All causes	2824	1371
Upper respiratory infections, cough	900	398
Otitis media	198	82
Lower respiratory infections	142	61
Enteritis, diarrhoea, vomiting	144	36
Specific infectious diseases	79	49
Conjunctivitis	87	26
Skin infections	38	41
Urinary infections	10	6
Unexplained fever	24	6
Rash	43	12
Dermatitis and eczema	116	28
Urticaria	12	10
Trauma	67	91
Asthma	9	12
Behavioural disorders	30	10
Sleep problems	10	1
Constipation	13	6
Enuresis	5	9

example of the influence of development on clinical presentation, an expanding intracranial lesion in a baby will cause an expanding head (hydrocephalus); but the same lesion in an older child or adult will cause the symptoms and signs of raised intracranial pressure.

It has been estimated that a British general practitioner with an average practice would see a new case of pyloric stenosis every 4 years, childhood diabetes every 6 years, Down's syndrome every 16 years, Turner's syndrome every 60 years and haemophilia or Hirschsprung's disease every 600 years! Hospitals, and especially teaching hospitals, give a very false impression of the pattern of illness in the community at large.

CHILDREN IN SOCIETY

The Registrar-General's five-point grading of social class is a crude but useful classification. Although it depends on the occupation of the father, we recognize that the father's occupation has close correlation with many other important factors including income, housing and attitudes to child rearing. In Britain the proportion of families in each social class is approximately:

I	Higher professional (usually university graduates)	6%
II	Other professional and technical	23%
III	Other non-manual and skilled manual	47%
IV	Semi-skilled manual	15%
V	Unskilled manual	5%

At least 4% of children cannot be classified because they do not have a parent with skills or employment. That "other" category constitutes an underclass which consistently fares less well than social class V (Table 1.1).

The health and educational progress of a child is directly related to the home and the environment. The child of an unskilled worker (social class V) has a 50% greater chance of being born dead or with a serious physical handicap than a lawyer's child (social class I). The disadvantage is there at birth and continues throughout childhood. The social class IV or V child will have more accidents, more physical illnesses, will be smaller and will read less well than the child from social class I or II.

Table 1.3. Social class and childhood mortality: death rates per 100 000. Death rates for younger children are more than twice as high as those of older children. At any age a child from social class V is twice as likely to die as one from social class I. In the age groups 5–9 and 10–14 about two-fifths of the deaths are due to accidents. From 1 to 4 years accidents are still the commonest cause of death followed in frequency by respiratory diseases, congenital abnormalities and neoplasms.

	Social class				
Age	I	II	III	IV	V
1–4	33	34	46	64	116
5–9	24	19	24	31	45
10–14	20	22	23	31	36

This class difference has remained much the same, or even widened, over the last 30 years despite overall improvements in mortality and morbidity rates, although in some respects social classes I–IV now resemble one another more closely while class V trails behind. Family size and birth order can also be important. The later children of large families tend to be smaller and have an increased chance of death in infancy or handicap later on.

Despite the fact that 25% of pregnancies are terminated, the proportion of children born outside marriage has risen to 27% of all births. About half of the children born outside marriage have parents who are living together, though not married, and are therefore likely to be brought up within a stable home. One-third of them are born to women under the age of 20 and many of those children stay with their mother or grandmother in what is often an unsatisfactory home. The change in the traditional pattern of family life and the increase in marital breakdown (1 in 3 ends in divorce) have resulted in about 15% of all families with children being single-parent families.

Unsatisfactory homes are not just those where there is overt cruelty, poverty or squalor. Stress at home may result from parental discord—quarrelling and separations, one-parent families, and children who have been put in the care of the wrong parent after divorce. It may result from parental illness—a dying or chronically handicapped mother, a mentally ill father, or just from parental inadequacy (work-shy parents, drunken parents and those who have given up the struggle of trying to be satisfactory parents).

The doctor sees the childhood casualties of these social events: poor development, illness and behavioural problems. Teachers see the casualties, too: unhappy children, delinquent children and children whose school progress is inappropriately slow.

The complexity and multiplicity of the factors that cause a child to be disadvantaged sometimes makes us feel helpless. However, since adversities compound one another, much may be achieved by modifying even one adverse factor. Even if we feel discouraged, it is worth trying to modify some aspects of the child's life to try to achieve at least one of the following factors.

1 Self-esteem (we need to feel wanted).
2 One good human relationship (we need to feel trusted).
3 Firm supervision and discipline (the game of life needs rules).

Extensive medical and social services exist, particularly for handicapped children, but all too often they are best used by well-informed, middle-class parents, while the parents of the disadvantaged child do not use them because either they do not know about them or they do not care. All medical and paramedical staff have a duty to recognize children in need or in distress and to see that they benefit from the help that is available.

COMMUNITY MEDICAL SERVICES

Health visitors

These are registered nurses who also hold a midwifery qualification and health visitor's certificate. They are employed by health authorities, but many are attached to group general practices and a few specialize (e.g. in diabetes) and have hospital attachments. They are responsible for family health, and particularly for mothers and young children. Their job is to prevent illness and handicap by giving appropriate advice, by detecting problems early and by mobilizing services to deal with those problems. They have an important role in health education.

Child health clinics

These clinics should be readily accessible to mothers with prams, and may be located in health centres, church or village halls, purpose-built accomodation or even in private houses. They are organized by health authorities and staffed by health visitors and doctors. Their role is a supervisory one. They offer routine medical and developmental examinations for infants and pre-school children, immunization, health education, and advice and support for those with special problems. About 90% of babies attend such a clinic during their first year but thereafter attendance falls off.

CHILD HEALTH SURVEILLANCE

The programme of health surveillance (Table 1.4) is a combined undertaking starting at birth with the hospital doctor or midwife and then involving the health visitor, general practitioner, clinical medical officer (at clinic or school) and school nurse. As the Department of Health itself points out, it cannot start too early for 'every effort should be made to ensure that women of child-bearing age are themselves healthy and that, by sensible family planning, pregnancies are welcome'.

Table 1.4. Child health surveillance.

Monitoring development
1 *Programme schedule*
(a) At birth. clinical examination (see p. 58) (doctor or midwife).
(b) At 6–10 days. Full clinical examination (doctor).
(c) 6 weeks. Assessment of well-being, weight gain and development (health visitor).
(d) 7–8 months. Review of development. Screening tests for vision and hearing (health visitor with medical back-up).
(e) 18 months. Review of development, especially social and language (health visitor). Opportunity to discuss toilet training.
(f) About 3 years. General review including hearing, vision, squint, teeth. Opportunity to discuss emotional and social problems.
(g) School entry. Comprehensive medical examination during first school year.
(h) School years. Regular checks of growth, hearing, vision, teeth. Testing of colour vision (especially boys) at 8–9 years. Examination of children about whom parents or teachers are concerned. Opportunities for older children to refer themselves to school doctor or nurse.

2 *Screening tests*
(a) Hearing and vision as above.
(b) Congenital dislocation of the hip—at birth. 6–10 days, 6 weeks.
(c) Phenylketonuria and hypothyroidism at 4–8 days.

Immunization
See p. 229

Health education and preparation for parenthood
During the final years at school and further education, and in the antenatal period, there are numerous opportunities for health education. As a contribution towards reducing child mortality and morbidity, the following matters deserve emphasis:
1 The dangers of delaying antenatal care.
2 The importance of good nutrition.
3 The adverse effects of smoking and of immoderate drinking during pregnancy upon the unborn baby.
4 The importance of fondling and talking to babies and of play.
5 The importance of breast feeding: the proper techniques of bottle feeding if the baby is not breast fed.
6 The relationship between parental smoking and respiratory disease in children.
7 How to recognize when a child is ill.
8 How to minimize the risks of accidents at home and on the road.
9 The importance of dental health.
10 The role of the father.

School health service

The school health service was established in 1904 because 40% of young men volunteering for service in the Boer War were found to be medically unfit. Today its main functions are to assess the state of health of schoolchildren, to help with the educational problems created by ill-health and to promote better health. The service is particularly important for children from unsatisfactory homes who may have missed out on pre-school health checks.

School medical officers are responsible, in conjunction with teachers, for identifying schoolchildren with disorders that are likely to interfere with their

Table 1.5. Incidence of some important problems.

At 1 year:
10% of boys have been circumcised

At 5 years:
7% have had at least one seizure
5% have a squint
5% have a behavioural problem
5% have a speech or language problem
2% have a substantial congenital defect

At 7 years:
16% have had tonsillectomy or adenoidectomy
13% require special education
10% wet their beds
10% have eczema, asthma or hay fever
2% have had a hernia repair
1% have had an appendicectomy

development, education and happiness, and for ensuring that they get whatever help they need.

Nursery schools

These may be separate schools or nursery classes attached to primary schools. They cater for children aged 3–5 years and are staffed by teachers specially trained in child development working with nursery nurses and assistants. They aim to encourage a child's development and learning by play, stimulation and physical activity. There is a widespread shortage of nursery school places, especially in industrial towns and cities. Priority is given to children with social or medical handicap and to those whose mothers need to go out to work.

Day nurseries

These are for pre-school children and cater for two main groups of children: those who require day-time care whilst their parents are at work or ill (particularly those who only have a single parent) and children from poor quality homes where stimulation and company are lacking. The number of day nurseries is few and the demand large. This has led to groups of parents forming their own centres for pre-school children, variously named *play groups*, play centres, crèches, etc. Most of these groups require considerable parent participation and organization and at present are mainly run by middle-class parents for their middle-class children.

SOCIAL SERVICES

The social services department of the local authority (not to be confused with the Department of Social Security, a central government department) is responsible for the care and/or supervision of children up to 18 years in a variety of circumstances: if they cannot be cared for by their parents or guardians temporarily or permanently, by reason of their illness or death, or because the children have been abandoned or lost. In certain circumstances the local authority may be designated a 'fit person' to assume parental rights in order to provide security and protection for the child.

Parental rights may be given to the local authority by the Court (usually the Juvenile Court), in which case a child is said to be the subject of a *care order*. The court must be satisfied that the child has suffered, or is likely to suffer, significant harm because of the standard of parental care or being beyond parental control. 'Harm' includes ill-treatment, sexual abuse, and the impairment of good physical and mental health and development.

The local authority tries to keep or place children with their own parents, relatives or friends whether care is temporary, permanent, voluntary or through a court order. When this is not possible local authority accommodation is used. It includes the following:

1   *Foster homes* in which a child is cared for in a family other than his own. Over half the children 'in care' are in foster homes; brief placements are successful, but long-term fostering tends to be unsuccessful. There are an increasing number of schemes in which the foster parents are paid additional money to look after children with physical and mental handicap or disturbed adolescents.

2   *Children's homes* are usually run on 'family' lines aiming to provide as normal an upbringing as possible, despite frequent changes of staff. They contain a higher proportion of difficult or handicapped children than foster homes. Of children in these homes, 95% still have a living parent, so that many are visited regularly or may be reunited with their parents for weekends or longer periods in the future. Children's homes are much more expensive for the local authority than fostering.

3   *Hostels for working children*.

4   *Residential nurseries*.

5   *Community homes* (formerly approved schools). Children may now be placed directly into these homes.

Children may be supervised in their own homes, either on a voluntary basis or as a result of a court *supervision order*. The social worker's prime aim here is to prevent family break-up and to try to help with problems of care, physical and emotional. The social worker is always glad to work as part of a team with others involved with the family, e.g. health visitors, doctors, teachers.

The social services department is also responsible for supervising children placed privately with foster parents. People who look after other people's children, whether on a day (child day-care, childminder) or residential (foster) basis, must register with their local social services department, even though they may be paid direct by the parent.

Children Act 1989

The Children Act (1989) is a major piece of legislation which repeals or substantially amends 55 earlier statutes. It affects all aspects of the welfare and protection of children including day-care, fostering and adoption, child abuse (pp. 241–2) and the consequences for children of marital breakdown. The spirit of the Act is reflected in the opening paragraphs. For example:

'the child's welfare shall be the court's paramount consideration'.

'any delay in determining the question (of the child's upbringing) is likely to pre-
   judice the welfare of the child'.

'a court shall have regard to . . . the ascertainable wishes and feelings of the child
   concerned'.

The concept of 'parental rights' is replaced by 'parental responsibilities'. If the
parents are married at the time of the child's birth, both have parental responsibilities. If they were not married, the mother has parental responsibility, but
there are legal mechanisms by which the father can acquire it.

Voluntary services

The statutory services are supplemented by a large number of voluntary and
charitable organizations, many of which were in existence before, and paved the
way for, statutory provisions. Many of those offering services to children have a
high level of professional expertise. The NSPCC (National Society for the
Prevention of Cruelty to Children) and its Scottish counterpart continue their
historic role of protecting children, and giving advice and support to families
under stress. Barnardos, the Children's Society and the National Children's
Homes have adapted their activities to the changing pattern of child needs. The
Save the Children Fund gives support to deprived inner cities in the UK as well
as relief in the Third World. Many voluntary bodies receive some funding from
central and/or local government.

Parent support groups now exist for almost every physical and mental
handicap and chronic disease of childhood (e.g. Spastics Society, Association for
Spina Bifida and Hydrocephalus, National Society for Mentally Handicapped
Children). Their membership consists largely of parents of affected children who
can offer advice to others from first-hand experience. They also raise money to
support research, thereby augmenting the work of the major medical research
charities (e..g. Action Research for the Crippled Child).

The Family Fund exists to give financial help to less well-off families with very
severely handicapped children. It is financed by the Department of Health but
administered by the Rowntree Trust in York. Charitable organizations can often
minimize bureaucracy and cut administrative costs and delays.

Adoption

Couples wishing to adopt a baby should approach either their local authority or
a registered adoption society. Each agency tends to have its own requirements,
for instance attachment to a particular religious denomination, or an age limit—it
is difficult to adopt a child if you are over 40. The agencies' main concern will be
relationships within the family, but it is also important for applicants to have a
steady income, a settled home and satisfactory health. Once accepted the
applicants have to wait anything from a few months to several years, until a
suitable baby is placed with them. A child of any age under 18 may be adopted
but the most usual placements are of illegitimate babies. The natural mother, and
in some circumstances the father, is asked to sign a form agreeing to the
adoption. There is a minimum 3 months' probationary period, during which the
natural mother can claim the baby back; about 2% do. During this period the

applicants will be visited by a social worker as will all the people concerned in the adoption. At the end of this time, if parental consents are signed and confirmed and reports on the adoptive home are satisfactory, the adoption order will be made in court. The child is now a full member of the adoptive family; he or she takes their name and has all the rights of a natural child (except that he or she cannot inherit a title!).

Medical examinations are required for both parents, for the baby before placement and again before the adoption hearing. It is essential to explain and discuss any suspected handicaps with the prospective parents. Parents are also advised to inform their child from the beginning that they are adopted and to explain this regularly and more fully as the child's understanding increases.

The availability of abortion, the increased tolerance shown by society to unmarried mothers, and the increased financial and practical support available for them have resulted in fewer babies being offered for adoption. There is now a shortage of healthy non-coloured babies for adoption, and an excess of childless couples wishing to adopt.

CHILDREN IN HOSPITAL

Until the middle of the 19th century the training of doctors and the provision of medical services (including hospitals) did not recognize the particular needs of children. In the following decades, when people like Charles Dickens and Lord Shaftesbury were stirring the public conscience to recognize the appalling circumstances in which many children grew up (or failed to do so), special hospitals for children began to be established. The first was in Liverpool (which also had the first organization in England for the prevention of cruelty to children) Eventually almost every city and large town had its children's hospital. The birth and development of paediatrics as a medical specialty was largely attributable to these hospitals, and they gave excellent service for a century or more.

In the later decades of the 20th century, the pattern of hospital care for children has changed. Children still have special needs—unrestricted visiting, facilities for resident mothers, play activities for younger children, education for the older—but the children's ward of today differs greatly from that of 30 years ago:

1 Child in-patients are, on average, much younger.
2 They are more severely ill.
3 They need all facilities for investigation and treatment.
4 The average stay in hospital is much shorter.
5 Parents are actively involved in care.
6 Many medical and surgical procedures are done as day-cases.
7 Neonatal care makes increasingly heavy demands on resources.

Although the number of children admitted to hospital has increased as new therapies have become available, their shorter stay in hospital means that fewer children's beds are needed. This, coupled with the need for access to expensive investigational technology, has resulted in the closure of all but a few large children's hospitals and the establishment of children's units in general hospitals.

Hospitals are not without risk to patients, especially child patients. The hazard of cross-infection is obvious: the hazard of mother–child separation is less obvious but can be more serious, especially among the 1–4-year olds. At this age children are old enough to grieve for a lost mother, but not old enough to understand the reason, or that the separation is temporary. 'Tomorrow' has no meaning for a toddler.

A young child separated from the mother may go through three stages:

1 Protest: he cries for her return.
2 Withdrawal: he curls up with a comfort blanket or toy and loses interest in food and play.
3 Denial: he appears happy, making indiscriminate friendships with everybody. This can be mistakenly interpreted as the child having 'settled', but the mother–child bond has been damaged and will have to be rebuilt. On returning home he may exhibit tantrums, refuse food or wet his bed.

These problems can be avoided or minimized by:

1 Avoiding hospital admission if possible.
2 Reducing the length of any admission to the minimum. Often the mother and family doctor can manage once the worst is over.
3 Performing operations (e.g. herniotomy, orchidopexy) and investigations (e.g. jejunal biopsy, colonoscopy) as day-cases.
4 Encouraging parents to visit often and arranging for one to sleep alongside a young child.

Hospital organization can also help to reduce stress. Children should be grouped together so that they may be looked after by staff specially trained and experienced in the care of children. Registered general nurses (RGN) usually see little of children during their training and need further experience if they are to hold senior posts on children's units. The same is true of occupational and physiotherapists. Teachers, nursery nurses and play leaders organize education and play. Segregation from adults allows children's wards to be less formal. The first impression of a children's ward should be of happy chaos rather than of the highly technical medicine which is in fact going on.

IMMIGRANT FAMILIES

The history of most countries involves the assimilation of new cultures and people from other lands, for man has always been a great traveller. The assimilation is usually gradual and in the early years beset with problems. Most countries today have immigrant communities with particular needs—the Vietnamese in Thailand, Moroccans and Turks in Belgium and the Indonesians in the Netherlands. In Britain, 5% of the population (and nearly 10% of the newborn) are of Asian or West Indian origin. Those figures disguise great regional variations from areas almost devoid of new commonwealth immigrants to others, such as Dewsbury and Bradford, where 30% of the newborn are of Pakistani origin. In Britain, the main medical problems and misunderstandings occur in relation to the large groups from the Indian subcontinent whose language and culture are poorly understood.

In general, particular sects of immigrants tend to live together, so that certain towns and cities may have a preponderance of one or other sect (e.g. Gujarati

Indians in Leicester and Pakistanis in Bradford). It is worth finding out if local immigrants are mainly of a particular sect or religion and to be aware of some of the differences. The main Asian groups are from:

1   North-east Pakistan and Bangladesh, usually Muslim (Islamic religion).
2   Gujarat in north-west India, mainly Hindu.
3   Punjab in northern India, usually Sikh.

There are several important medical aspects which are discussed below.

1   Names

Selecting the appropriate and polite name can be difficult. Sikh boys have the complementary name Singh, and girls Kaur. The personal name precedes the complementary name and the subcaste name (surname) follows it, e.g. Davindar Kaur Bhumbra. The Hindu naming system is somewhat similar. Devi for girls and Lal for boys are common complementary names, and may be joined on to the first personal name, e.g. Arima Devi Chopra becomes Arimadevi Chopra. Some Sikhs and Hindus will not use a subcaste name. Muslim names are more difficult; often there is no shared family name. Males have a religious title (e.g. Mohammed or Abdul) which may precede or follow the personal name. Females have a title (e.g. Begum or Bibi) and a personal name. It is discourteous to use the religious name or title on its own; it must be coupled with the personal name. (In close friendship the personal name is used on its own without the religious name or title.)

2   Contact with foreign diseases

Most children will have been born and brought up in Britain. But if the child has recently arrived in the country, or returned from visiting relatives in the parents' homeland, he or she is at risk of unusual illnesses (malaria is seen in children returning from Pakistan and hookworm in those from tropical and subtropical regions) and diseases that are more common abroad (e.g. tuberculosis in India and Pakistan).

3   Racial susceptibility to disease

Some diseases are exclusive to certain races, e.g. sickle-cell disease in negroes. More commonly a disease is simply more likely in particular races, e.g. thalassaemia major which is common in Pakistanis, and very common in Cypriots. The indigenous British white is more likely to be born with cystic fibrosis or spina bifida, and is particularly susceptible to refractive errors —spectacles are part of the national uniform for the over forties. Consanguinity (marrying a blood relative) is common in some cultures, particularly Muslims. The offspring have an increased chance of receiving the same recessive gene from each parent, and of developing an otherwise rare genetically determined disease.

4   Food

Asian families are prone to nutritional problems because of the difficult compromise they have to achieve between their religious beliefs and the British food industry. Orthodox Hindus are vegetarian, less strict Hindus avoid beef, and any food which has been processed with utensils that may have been in contact with beef. Muslims avoid pork with similar strictness, and any meat must be killed in a special way (Halal). Muslim children at puberty may join the Ramadan month-long fast each year. Although Asians are considerable users of butter, they will not use margarine (which is a notable source of vitamin D for many British families).

5 Customs

Asian women avoid exposure to sunlight; vitamin D deficiency is common in pregnancy and is a risk for their newborn babies. As the girls reach puberty they adopt traditional clothes which shield their limbs and skin from sunlight; the chance of rickets is increased. Orthodox Muslim women are relatively confined to the home, and lead a restricted life; very often the husband will be responsible for all outside activities including taking the child to a doctor or hospital. The person accompanying the child to the clinic may be the most senior male member of the family or the best at speaking English, yet know little of the child's problem or the mother's worries. Parents who themselves were brought up and educated in a developing country may have old-fashioned beliefs about health, and often have no recognition that emotional factors may cause or exacerbate pain.

The cumulative effect of these social and cultural factors is important for the child from conception and through school. Thus the Muslim mother in Britain compared with her white neighbours is more likely to be in social class V, to conceive before the age of 15 or after the age of 35, to have more than four children, to have less antenatal care, more anaemia and a baby of low birth weight. The rates for stillbirth, infant death and major congenital abnormalities are twice as great, and the chance of the child requiring special education even greater. Enquiring about the racial background or the family cultural and religious beliefs should not be a source of embarrassment; nor is it a basis for unfair discrimination. In practice we behave as if all children are born equal—then we respect and cater for their differences and difficulties. We want an aristocracy of achievement.

LAWS RELATING TO THE YOUNG

For legal purposes a child remains a 'child' up to the age of 14, is a 'young person' up to 17, and is an adult at 18. However, many laws become operative at other ages.

School

School education is compulsory for children aged 5 and over. Children may not leave until they are 16.

Work

Children may not be employed until they are 13. Then they may be employed only between the hours of 7 am and 7 pm, and for a maximum of 2 hours on school days.

Abuse

It is an offence to:

Tattoo anyone under 18.

Seduce a girl under 16.

Sell tobacco to a child under 16.

Sell fireworks to a child under 13.

Expose to fire risk (e.g. not use a fire guard) a child under 12.

Give intoxicating liquor to children under 5.

Crime

Children under 10 (under 8 in Scotland) are not considered 'criminally responsible' for their misdeeds, and may be dealt with by Juvenile Courts.

The court can make (1) a 'Care Order' giving parental rights to the local authority, or (2) a 'Supervision Order' which may be administered by the social services department or, if the child is over 14, by the probation department. At the age of 15 children can be sent to Borstal.

Adult courts deal with those over the age of 17. Although it is legally possible to be sent to prison for a first offence at the age of 17, it is in practice rare before the age of 20.

At the age of 100 the child may receive a telegram of congratulation from the Queen.

FURTHER READING

Forfar JO. *Child Health in a Changing Society*. Oxford University Press.

Mitchell RG. *Child Health in the Community*. Churchill Livingstone.

Henley A. *Asian Patients in Hospital and at Home*. Kings Fund Publishing Office.

Qureshi BA. *Transcultural Medicine—Dealing with Patients from Different Cultures*. Kluwer Academic Publishers.

Chapter 2
Parents and Children:
Listening and Talking

When compared with other animal species, *Homo sapiens* takes an inordinate length of time to achieve independence from parents. Through most of childhood, therefore, parents must act as intermediaries between child-patient and doctor. Parents tell us about the child's symptoms, although the children contribute more and more as they grow older. Similarly parents put into effect any treatments needed outside hospital.

Small children only survive because their parents are concerned about them. A few are less concerned than they should be and their children suffer from neglect. Others are more than usually concerned. Doctors tend to refer to them as anxious or over-anxious and they may be regarded as a nuisance, forever cluttering a busy GP's surgery. These different patterns often reflect the parents' own upbringing, as do excessive concerns with physiological functions, such as eating, sleeping and bowel habits.

Most parents also want their children to succeed—to be above average in height and intelligence, to be at least in the top half and preferably in the top 10%. Some parents want their children to succeed in fields that are important to them, such as sport; some want them to help with, and later take over, a family business; most wish for their children achievements or material possessions that they themselves had to manage without.

Paediatric history taking is therefore complex and often time-consuming. The doctor must try to disentangle the factual account from parental interpretations and overtones. 'He has vomited 3 times', 'He has had a rash' or 'He gets wheezy when he runs about' are factual statements. 'The baby has colic', 'He is lazy at school' or 'He is not eating properly' are interpretations. 'He was feverish' usually means his skin felt hot, not that a raised temperature was recorded.

HISTORY-TAKING

The child's history covers the same ground as that of an adult patient, with some important additions. We need to know the name, sex and date of birth of the child, and the name of the school, nursery, clinic or health centre he attends. Ask what the child is called at home and use that name. Address the parents as 'Mr and Mrs Jackson', not as 'Mother' or 'Dad'. The conversation will be more productive if everyone is at ease. A young child may be happiest on a parent's knee. A more independent one may have more fun playing with toys which should be available. An older child must be fully included in the discussion. Arrange the furniture to encourage a sense of partnership between parents and doctor. Avoid confrontation over the top of a desk.

It is usually best to start with the history of the *presenting symptoms* because this is what they have come to tell you about. Let them tell it their own way first; then ask specific questions to fill in necessary details. Frequent interruptions or insistence on ordered chronology will inhibit free speech. Like any other work of art, a clinical history is rarely perfect at the first attempt. Practice receiving histories as well as taking them. If the problem is not an acute one, it is important to find out how the illness is affecting the child's life. School is the equivalent of an adult's employment. How much school has been missed through illness? Has the child opted out of games or of leisure activities at home? Ask about patterns of eating, sleeping and activity. If these have not changed, serious illness is unlikely. A diminution in appetite or activity, or an increased need for sleep, are likely to be significant. Recorded weight loss is always important.

Ask for the parents' own ideas about what is the matter with the child. Sometimes it will enable you to assuage an unnecessary anxiety; at other times it may lead to a correct diagnosis you had not considered. Mothers are more likely than anyone else to understand their babies' cries, and research shows that babies can 'talk'. They have different cries for hunger, pain, etc.; and the characteristic cries of meningitis, Down's syndrome and hypothyroidism are all different. The mother will usually know when the cry is abnormal and sometimes will be able to suggest a reason.

It is often helpful, especially if psychological problems are suspected, to ask 'What kind of boy (girl) is he (she)?' The answer may be 'a worrier', 'placid', 'never still', 'obsessional'. If you then ask 'Who does he takes after?', it often provides useful insight for the parent. It is also helpful to know what the child does in his spare time and whether he is by nature gregarious or solitary.

Previous medical history should include not only details of bad illnesses, operations or hospital attendances, but also any allergies or drug sensitivities. It is worth remembering that a history of rubella is extremely unreliable: many other minor infections simulate rubella. The immunization history must be included; it may help to exclude a suspected condition, and it identifies those families in need of advice about further immunization. Diphtheria/tetanus/pertussis vaccine is often referred to as triple vaccine or 3-in-1, but since the introduction of measles/mumps/rubella vaccine it may be wise to avoid these potentially confusing phrases. Many mothers will have their child's parents-held health record which includes details of previous weights, immunizations and other health events. Children are normally weighed and measured during their first year at school.

The *family history* should include the following.

1 The ages of the siblings and parents.
2 Whether any other member of the family has or has had the same condition as the child, whether it be a rash and fever (? has the child caught the same infection), or six digits on each hand (? has the child an inherited condition that runs in the family).
3 What illnesses the parents and close relatives have had, in order to allay needless worries. The parents may worry that their child's stomach ache is caused by stomach cancer, because a relative recently died with it.
4 An enquiry regarding consanguinity, especially in Muslim families, because rare inherited conditions are more likely if the parents are related.

The *perinatal history* should provide details of the pregnancy, birth and first week of life. In the pregnancy, establish its length (normal is 40 weeks) and any maternal infections, illnesses, or abnormalities. Details of the delivery should include the place of birth, presentation (head or breech), type (spontaneous, forceps or caesarean section) and the birth weight. Any abnormality of the neonatal period is soon discovered by asking if the baby needed special care (in an incubator, or an intensive care unit) after birth. A healthy baby would have been allowed to be with his mother for the first day, and be allowed home with his mother at the planned time. Slowness to feed in the early days and cyanotic or apnoeic attacks are sometimes indicators of brain damage.

The *developmental history* is almost unique to paediatrics. It is important, particularly for young or handicapped children. It includes details of the times at which skills such as walking and talking were acquired (full details in Chapter 3).

The *social history* is obtained, after establishing rapport with the parents, by talking with them about their life, their home, their work and their problems. Find out the father's job (it is a useful financial guide), and find out exactly what the job entails; a 'lorry driver' may be a local parcel deliverer or a long-distance lorry driver who is away from home much of the time. Does the mother go out to work and, if so, who looks after the child? If the mother is now a housewife, what was her job before? If she was a nurse, she will have a different level of knowledge and a different need for information. Three particular areas must be explored which have a direct influence on the child's development:

1   The family composition: are the mother and father living together? If so, in harmony or discord? Or is this a single-parent family?
2   The financial situation: is the family financially viable, with a regular income, or are they dependent on social security grants?
3   Housing: have they a home of their own, and if so, what sort? Or are they living with relatives or in a hostel? Satisfactory housing should have not more than 1.5 persons per room, a supply of hot water and indoor sanitation.

We each find some parents easy to interview, and others difficult. It is as well to get into the habit of blaming ourselves if the history is unclear. If you are tempted to label someone a 'bad historian', remember that a historian is the person who collects and records the history!

When the history has been taken and the examination of the child completed (Chapter 3) the family will be waiting anxiously for the doctor's 'verdict.' Their fears are usually far worse than the reality. At this point the doctor will probably know enough to point the conversation in one of three directions:

1   Explanation and reassurance.
2   The need for investigation and/or treatment but with a favourable outcome probable.
3   Bad news.

Reassurance is readily accepted by some parents who 'just wanted to make sure everything was all right'. An experienced doctor may detect that the child's condition was only a pretext to visit him, and that more serious concerns lie elsewhere. Others are very difficult to reassure. Patient explanation is usually helpful. People rarely stop worrying because somebody says, 'Don't worry'. They may stop if they fully understand why the doctor is not worried. A specific anxiety needs an equally specific reassurance. Thus, if parents fear that their child's pallor may be due to leukaemia, a normal blood count may be insufficient reassurance. They need to hear the doctor say. 'He has not got leukaemia'.

Investigations and treatments must be explained in advance to parents and to children old enough to understand. Very few investigations in children need overnight hospital admission. Simple things can be done at an outpatient visit. Multiple or complex tests can often be planned within a day on the ward. Be honest. Many blood tests require a needle in a vein, and that is painful. A CT brain scan is noisy (or, for babies and very young children, may require a general anaesthetic). Children are very forgiving if you are honest with them.

Parents want to know the results of tests, and their implications, as soon as possible. Do not keep them waiting unnecessarily.

Treatments to be given by parents must be explained and reasons given (e.g. why 4 times a day?). Techniques for the use of inhalers for asthma, injections for diabetes or rectally administered anticonvulsants must be demonstrated.

Today's parents are far more informed about medical matters than were their parents, principally from television programmes and newspaper and magazine articles. Unfortunately the media tend to exaggerate or sensationalize, presenting an experimental new treatment as a 'breakthrough', or a particular clinic or hospital (often in another country) as 'the only one of its kind' and hence by implication, the best. The accolade of a TV hype is more impressive than holy writ, and the doctor trying to put things in perspective may have an uphill task. We need special understanding for parents who have been offered hope when they had none before.

Bad news in paediatrics is usually:
1   The recognition of a serious birth defect in a newborn baby.
2   The recognition of a serious handicap in a young child.
3   The diagnosis of a serious, progressive or incurable disease.

The news that a baby is deformed is a great shock to the parents. Even minor anomalies are seen as major tragedies. At the first interview detailed explanations will not be grasped. If the baby is to be transferred to another hospital for early surgery, the mother must have a chance to see her infant before removal. She will need frequent progress reports on the baby until she is able to visit. The closer the contact the parents maintain with the baby, the less likely are they to reject it if there is a residual handicap. If the baby survives, the parents need patient explanation of the care needed and how to recognize any problems that are likely to arise. Parents of children with serious defects or handicaps will need advice about the recurrence risks if they plan another child later on. For easily recognizable conditions in which a genetic (or non-genetic) basis is clearly established, the family doctor or paediatrician can provide this information. For more complex problems reference to a *genetic counselling* clinic is advisable. The three basic essentials for counselling are:
1   A firmly established diagnosis, which is often more difficult than it sounds.
2   A full family history.
3   Ample time to elicit facts and anxieties, and to explain recurrence risks, prenatal tests and other relevant issues.

All this implies ready access to doctors and nurses who can listen and answer, and who can at least give the apperance of having unlimited time to spare. Parents of seriously handicapped children can often help one another through membership of parents' associations or organizations.

In summary, whenever serious disease is diagnosed in a child parents want to know:

1   Exactly what is the matter, in terms they can grasp.
2   What the doctors can do about it.
3   What the parents can do about it.
4   The outlook for this child.
5   The outlook for any other children that may follow.
6   Why it happened, but this cannot always be answered.

Parents' reactions to bad news tends to follow a recognizable pattern, although the time-scale varies widely from one family to another (Fig. 2.1). It is important to recognize this, not only for the purposes of helping, but so that the doctor is not hurt by finding himself the target of parental anger, or irritated by the difficulties of communication. The stages of adaptation to personal tragedy, which often overlap, are as follows.

1   Intellectual and emotional numbness. Information does not get in. Emotions do not get out. The doctor may be relieved that the parents have 'taken it so well'. He may later be annoyed if parents say 'nobody told us anything' when he spent hours telling them everything.

2   Denial. The message has got through but cannot yet be believed. 'There must be some mistake' or 'But he will catch up, won't he?' are characteristic of this stage. The doctor must resist the temptation to hedge or to use woolly phrases such as 'slow developer' which encourage parents to believe that the problem is temporary.

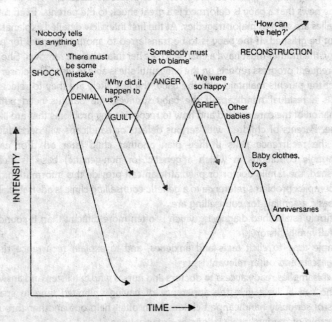

Fig. 2.1. Emotional response to bad news.

3   Guilt and anger. Now the truth has registered and blame must be apportioned. Parents usually blame themselves for some act of commission or omission, real or imaginary. The feeling of guilt may be so intolerable that they need to blame somebody else, personal (the doctor) or impersonal (the tablets).

4   All being well, this is followed by grieving, which is a natural and healing process. Tears are appropriate, and if they are shed in the presence of the doctor he or she should not be embarrassed. They represent a privileged communication and tell the doctor that the final stage is near.

5   Reconstruction. The former pattern of family life has been demolished. The new must now be built. It is imperative that the parents are given a key, active role in any therapeutic programme. Never say 'Nothing can be done'.

Does he take sugar?

This phrase was the title of a TV series about mentally handicapped people, to illustrate how easy it is to talk about people in their presence as if they were not there. It is a risk faced by all children (and elderly people), not just mentally handicapped people. Children from about 2 years on can hear, understand and say a lot. By 7 or 8, they are wise. Don't talk about them as if they had no understanding—and you may have to discourage parents from doing the same. Many doctors who commence the consultation talking with both parent and child together conclude by talking with each privately—'Please will you wait outside whilst I talk with your mother and then I will ask her to wait outside whilst I talk with you: so that will be fair to everyone'.

As children with chronic illness approach adolescence, parents find it particularly difficult to loosen the apron-strings. The doctor can make a small contribution by treating young teenagers as equal with parents during consultations, and, as they get older, by talking principally with the young patient.

By the same token, whatever the medical problem, the child is first a child. Not 'he is a diabetic' or 'she is an epileptic': he has diabetes, she has epilepsy.

Finally, do not, in conversation with parents, refer to their baby as 'it'. If in doubt, better to risk an incorrect 'he' or 'she' than render their infant sexless.

Chapter 3
Examination of Children*

The prospect of examining children, especially the very young, for the first time is often daunting to students, but children are usually the most cooperative of patients and clinical examination should be a happy experience for them. All but the oldest will be accompanied by one or more adults who can be a real help to the doctor and thereby feel involved in the exercise and not just spectators.

The approach will, of course, vary according to the child's age. Examination of babies at birth (see p. 58) and in the early weeks of life requires patience, warm hands and a quiet voice: bedside manner contributes little. From the age of 2–3 months, babies respond to friendly advances and some degree of rapport—even cooperation—can be established. Around 6 months of age babies are indiscriminately friendly towards everybody so examination is easy, but by 10 months and through toddlerhood children may be suspicious of strangers. Their confidence can be won, perhaps by the offering and accepting of something to hold, but not in a hurry.

These young children present the biggest challenge to the doctor. They dislike being separated from their parents and they do not like being made to lie flat, so examination on mother's knee or standing close beside her is often more profitable than putting the child on an examination couch. Some children (not only adolescents) are reluctant to remove clothes. The doctor must therefore be patient and adaptable—neither the pace nor the order of the examination can be dictated by the doctor.

By school age (5 years) children have become used to being without their parents (though many prefer them to be nearby in the unfamiliar surroundings of surgery or clinic) and to doing what they are asked (by and large). The apprehensive child can usually be diverted by small-talk. As childhood advances, therefore, clinical examination comes to resemble the pattern for adults.

There are at least two distinct purposes in clinical examination. One is to seek abnormal signs as an aid to diagnosis. In acute illnesses of early childhood symptoms are often non-specific, so important signs (infected throat, stiff neck or infected urine) will be missed if the doctor does not look for them systematically. The other is as a basis for reassurance. A 'thorough examination' is a powerful therapeutic weapon if the problem is inappropriate parental axiety. Parents do not readily accept reassurance if the doctor has not examined the child (and quite right, too).

* To augment the description of clinical examination in Chapter 3, a 30-minute videotape, Clinical Examination of Children, has been produced and is available from University Audiovisual Service, University of Leeds, Leeds LS2 8JT.

PHYSICAL GROWTH

The characteristics of children which most clearly distinguish them from adults are growth (increase in size) and development (increase in complexity and the acquisition of new skills).

Growth is traditionally estimated by weight and height (length in babies). Rates of increase are good indicators of general health and nutrition. Other useful measurements include sitting height (which reflects body proportions, Fig. 3.1), span (which is usually similar to height) and skin-fold thickness (which measures fat). Growth is rapid in the first year and at puberty but remarkably constant between.

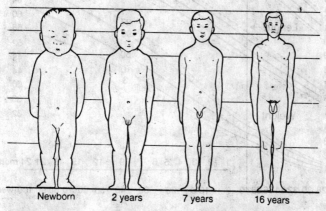

Newborn   2 years   7 years   16 years

Fig. 3.1. Body proportions from birth to adulthood. The ratio of the parts above and below the symphysis pubis falls from 1.7 : 1 in the newborn to 0.9 : 1 in the adult.

Children should be weighed either in underclothes (babies in nappies) or naked, but always the same way because changes in weight are more important than absolute values. Height and length can be most accurately measured with stadiometers which are expensive. If children are upset at the prospect of being weighed and measured, leave it until the clinical examination is over. Tears are more easily prevented than stopped.

Height, weight and head circumference can best be interpreted by reference to centile charts or tables (Fig. 3.2, Table 3.1). Centile charts are constructed from measurements of many children who reach their pubertal growth spurts at different ages. At puberty the growth curve for an individual child will first accelerate towards a higher centile, then gradually level off towards final height. Height charts need to be interpreted in conjunction with pubertal status (p. 25) and bone age (p. 26).

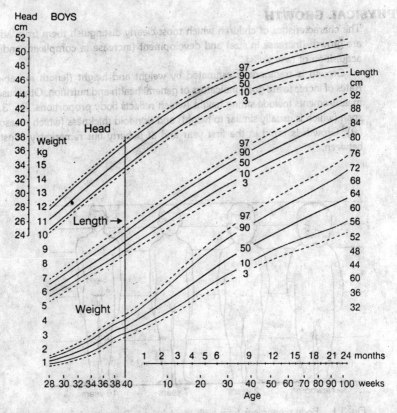

Fig. 3.2. A growth record (centile chart) for head circumference, length (height) and weight. Similar charts are available for various age ranges for each sex.

Table 3.1. Head circumference (cm) centile table.

	3%	50%	97%
Birth	33	35	38
12 months	43	47	49
18 months	45	49	51
2 years	46	50	52
3 years	47	50	53
5 years	48	51	54
8 years	50	52	55
12 years	51	54	56
14 years	52	56	58

Dental development

The average ages of eruption of the teeth are shown in Table 3.2 but there is a wide normal range (see p. 161).

Table 3.2 Teeth. There are 20 deciduous and 32 permanent teeth. Permanent teeth appear from the 6th year. The first molars and central incisors appear first. All teeth have appeared by the age of 14 except the third molars. Teeth appear a few months earlier in girls.

Deciduous		Appearance (months)
Central incisor	lower	6–10
	upper	7–10
Lateral incisor	upper	8–10
	lower	12–18
First molar		12–18
Canine		16–20
Second molar		20–30

SEXUAL DEVELOPMENT

Human sexual development is concentrated into two relatively brief periods of time. Primary sexual differentiation takes place from the 6th week of embryonic life. The gonad, which is undifferentiated up to this time, develops into a testicle in the presence of a Y chromosome or into an ovary in the presence of two X chromosomes. The gonad then produces fetal hormones which influence the development of the Wolffian and Müllerian systems (gonaducts) along appropriate lines. The external genitalia develop a female pattern unless there are fetal androgens to masculinize them (Fig. 3.3).

Secondary sex characteristics develop at puberty in response to pituitary gonadotrophins. The trigger which releases these hormones is still unknown. The age of onset of puberty is very variable, being influenced by racial, hereditary and nutritional factors. In Britain today breast development begins at 11 years on average, pubic hair a little later and menstruation at 13, but ranging from 9 to 17 years: boys mature a little later. In both sexes, puberty is accompanied by an impressive growth spurt, which is maximal in girls at the age of 12 and in boys at 14. Breast development in girls and growth of the testes and penis in boys are

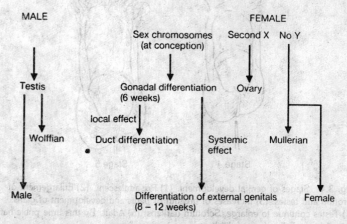

Fig. 3.3. Normal sex differentiation.

usually the first signs of puberty. Early breast development may be asymmetrical. Gonadal hormones are chiefly responsible for these changes, but adrenal androgens play a part. The progress of puberty may be recorded in relation to the stages of pubic hair (both sexes), external genitalia (males), and breast development (Fig. 3.4 and 3.5). Epiphyseal fusion, with cessation of growth, marks the end of puberty.

Bone age (or skeletal age) is a useful index of growth and is determined from X-rays, of the hand and wrist at most ages, though the knee and foot are helpful in small babies. The bones and epiphyses calcify, and hence become visible on X-rays, in a regular order. Later the epiphyses fuse in a similar regular fashion. X-rays can be compared with age-related standards (as in the Greulich and Pyle atlas, which is widely used but is based on American children and is up to 2.5 years out for British children): or it can be scored by more complex methods such as the British Tanner and Whitehouse scheme. Neither method is very accurate and great care is needed in interpreting scores. In healthy children bone age

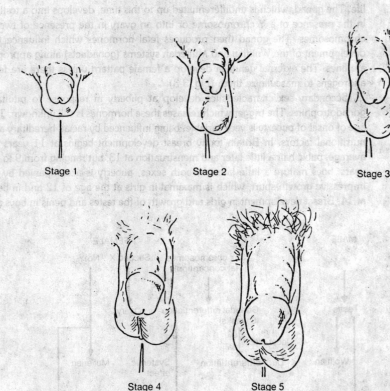

Stage 1

Stage 2

Stage 3

Stage 4

Stage 5

Fig. 3.4 Stages of genital development. (1) Pre-adolescent. (2) Enlargement of scrotum and testes. (3) Increases of breadth of penis and development of glans. (4) Testes continue to enlarge. Scrotum darkens. (5) Adult. By this time pubic hair has spread to medial surface of thighs.

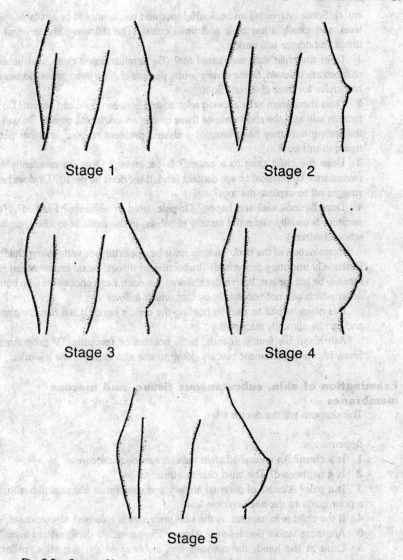

Fig. 3.5. Stages of breast development. (1) Pre-adolescent—elevation of papilla only. (2) Breast bud stage. (3) Further enlargement of breast and areola. (4) Projection of areola and papilla above level of breast. (5) Mature stage—areola has recessed, papilla projects.

relates more closely to height than to age, short children tending to have 'delayed', and tall children 'advanced' bone ages.

GENERAL EXAMINATION

Whilst the doctor is listening to the clinical history he will be learning a lot about the child and the relationships between the child and the accompanying parent(s). Some interesting and colourful toys and books should be available at low level, and ideally a low table and small chairs. The following are amongst the things the doctor will notice.

1 Does the child look well cared for? (Be careful. Some clean, well-behaved children are unloved. Some caring young parents choose outrageous clothes and hair-styles for their children) So . . .

2 Does there seem to be a loving relationship between child and parent? Do the parents talk as if the child was not there or was an inanimate object? Do you get the feeling that they have brought a shared problem to you? Is either parent trying to opt out?

3 Does the child cling to a parent? Is he crying? Does he constantly seek reassurance by physical or eye contact (and, if so, does he get it)? Or does he go straight off to explore the toys?

4 Does he look well and happy? Or pale, tired or unhappy? Flushed? (Temperature is usually measured rectally in babies, in the axilla in toddlers, orally in schoolchildren.)

Examination of the body systems must be opportunistic with young children. Potentially upsetting procedures (inspection of throat, rectal examination) may sensibly be left for last. With older children the doctor can choose his own batting order which will not necessarily be that which follows.

It is often helpful to start by holding the child's hand. It is a friendly gesture and can be clinically informative.

Ask about his family, friends, pets, hobbies or favourite TV programmes. Show him any instrument you are going to use and explain how it works.

Examination of skin, subcutaneous tissue, and mucous membranes

The *skin* can tell the doctor a lot.

Appearance:

1 Is it clean? An unwashed child indicates inadequate care.

2 Is it pigmented? The chief clue to ethnic origin.

3 Is it pale? A cause of parental anxiety and sometimes a sign of ill-health, but a poor guide to the haemoglobin level.

4 If the child is in nappies, is the skin underneath inflamed or excoriated?

5 Are there visible skin lesions? A rash? Pigmented or depigmented areas?

6 Look at the hands for cyanosis and clubbing of the fingertips, pallor or abnormal creases on the palms.

Feel:

1 Is it rough and dry? This is most commonly indicative of an atopic constitution.

2 Is it inelastic? Pinch up a fold of skin (not fat), then let go. A slow recoil indicates dehydration.

The most important *subcutaneous organs* are fat and lymph glands. *Fat* is a useful guide to nutritional state. An undernourished child is 'all skin and bone'.

The limbs are slender, the buttocks flat, the bony prominences conspicuous. Excess fat is most evident on the trunk. Fat can be measured with skin-fold calipers. Mid upper-arm circumference (MUAC) can be measured quickly and cheaply. In children aged 1–5 years, a circumference less than 14 cm suggests poor nutrition and needs further assessment. If there has been recent weight loss, the skin of the lower abdomen and inner aspects of the thighs are like a puppy's neck.

Superficial lymph glands are always palpable in the neck and groins of children, and sometimes in the axilla. Normal glands are soft, mobile, non-tender and usually not larger than an acorn. Enlarged tonsillar glands, just behind the angle of the jaw, indicate past or present throat infections. Generalized lymphadenopathy suggests systemic illness unless it is due to widespread skin disease (e.g. infantile eczema).

The mucous membranes, especially of the eye, tongue and lips, are a fair guide to moderate or severe anaemia but not to lesser degrees of anaemia. It is particularly important to examine them in coloured children: their skin pigment disguises their pallor. The assessment of minor degrees of jaundice is not possible in some forms of artificial lighting. Any reasonable suspicion of anaemia or jaundice should prompt appropriate blood tests.

Examination of the fontanelles and head circumference
The *fontanelles* of the infant's skull are God's gift to paediatricians. The *anterior* fontanelle is wide open at birth and gradually becomes smaller. By 6 months of age it is about 3 × 4 cm; by 1 year it is the size of a finger tip; by 1.5 years it has usually closed. Gentle pressure over the fontanelle gives an indication of its tension. It pulsates in time with the heart beat.
A *large* fontanelle usually means hydrocephalus.
A *small* fontanelle usually means slow brain growth.
A *sunken* fontanelle usually means dehydration.
A *bulging* fontanelle in a child who is not crying usually means raised intracranial pressure.

The *posterior* fontanelle is far back where the sagittal and lambdoid sutures meet. It closes soon after birth.

A *third* fontanelle is sometimes present in the sagittal suture between the anterior and posterior fontanelles. It closes with the anterior fontanelle. It may be mistaken for a late-closing posterior fontanelle.

The *head circumference* is an important measurement, especially in the first 2 years of life when it is increasing rapidly. It reflects the volume of the cranial contents with surprising accuracy. Abnormalities of fontanelle size and tension in apparently healthy babies should be interpreted against a background of serial measurements of head circumference (i.e. *rate* of growth: see also p. 115).

The circumference to be measured is the biggest, so the tape measure (good quality, inelastic) should pass over the occiput, above the ears and over the prominence of the brow, and it is wise to take two or three measurements in slightly different planes to establish the biggest. The measurement should be recorded on a centile chart (Fig. 3.2, p. 24).

Examination of the neuromuscular system

The younger the child, the less a neurological examination will resemble the traditional pattern used for adults. As with developmental examination, much will be learned about the child's *functional* abilities and difficulties by watching him play. Is his mobility appropriate for his age? Does he seem to have any difficulties with coordination, vision or hearing? Is he unsteady (ataxic) on his legs? Does he use both sides of his body well? Is hand dominance established (it seldom is under 2 years)?

In young children with cerebral palsy, mental handicap, muscular dystrophy and some progressive disorders, formal neurological examination adds little to observations of function, although hearing and vision will need to be carefully tested. In older children with acute neurological disease (tumour, abscess, intracranial haemorrhage) clinical examination helps to localize the lesion and to indicate what further investigations are needed.

Primitive reflexes (responses)

These reflexes are present in early life but disappear as myelination is completed and cortical control develops. They vary in intensity during the early months, start to go from 3 months and should be gone by 6 months. A strongly positive primitive reflex after 6 months indicates cerebral damage. Examples of such primitive reflexes are:

1   The Moro reflex which occurs in response to many stimuli. One method of eliciting it is to hold the baby supine with the head supported in one hand. When the head is allowed to drop 5 cm (2 inches) onto the other hand, there is sudden extension and abduction of the upper limbs, with opening of the hands, followed by flexion to the midline. The movement should be symmetrical.

2   The plantar and palmar grasp reflexes, in which fingers or toes flex in response to a finger being pressed on the palm or sole respectively, and are released by pressure along the extensor surface of the fingers or toes.

3   Asymmetrical tonic neck reflex. As the infant turns his head to the side, the limbs on the chin side extend and those on the occipital side flex. This reflex is maximal at the age of 3 months.

General neurological assessment

Assessment of *muscle tone* is important. If an infant or young child has generalized hypotonia, the legs can be flexed on the trunk so that the feet are by the ears without discomfort. If the child is picked up under the arms, the shoulders tend to rise up towards the ears. Hypertonia (spasticity) usually results in the elbows being flexed and the knees extended. The thigh adductors are often involved, causing the extended legs to cross. It may be difficult to distinguish true spasticity from voluntary contraction of muscles, but spasticity is usually accompanied by other signs of an upper motor neurone lesion.

Muscle power is best tested in children old enough to cooperate by giving simple commands, e.g. 'squeeze my fingers', 'push me away'.

Tendon reflexes are normally brisk in the legs but may be more difficult to elicit in the arms. Reinforcement will often help to demonstrate an apparently absent reflex.

The *plantar response* should be elicited from the lateral aspect of the sole, moving the stimulus from the front to the back. It is normally extensor until the child starts walking. Stimulation of the anterior part of the sole in young babies will elicit the plantar grasp reflex in which all the toes curl down.

Ankle clonus, if sustained, is suggestive of an upper motor neurone lesion. It is best tested for with the knee semi-flexed. Dorsiflex the ankle sharply, trying different degrees of pressure. Pressing too lightly or too hard may mask clonus.

Coordination may be tested in children more than 2 years old by the finger–nose and heel–shin manoeuvres. In younger children it is more helpful to watch for any unsteadiness when playing. A 3-year-old can stand on one leg briefly, and make a good attempt to walk heel-to-toe along a straight line on the floor.

To test for *dysdiadochokinesis*, ask the child to copy you patting the back of one hand as fast as possible, and then the other. Even 10-year-olds cannot do it as fast as an adult can.

Examination of cranial nerves

The *fundi* should not be difficult to see in older children. Ask the child to look at something across the room and keep your head out of the line of vision. Dim room lighting will result in the patient's and the doctor's pupils dilating, but make sure the ophthalmoscope light is bright. In younger children cooperation cannot be obtained. Attempts to force the eyelids apart will provoke strong opposition. Mydriatic eye drops (e.g. tropicamide) and patience, with or without sedation, usually prevail. Breast- or bottle-fed infants can often be examined during a feed. If detailed examination of the fundi is necessary it may have to be done under anaesthesia.

Visual fields can be tested in older children by the confrontation technique, though they find it difficult to keep their gaze fixed. In babies, their attention can be attracted by one person sitting face-to-face whilst the tester, standing behind the baby, advances an object from the periphery of the field.

Eye movements can be tested from about 3 months by getting the child to fix on a bright or colourful object and then slowly moving it in each direction whilst gently restraining head movements.

Squint (strabismus) may be obvious. It is usually a convergent squint of one or both eyes secondary to a defect of visual acuity (concomitant squint) in a young child. If of recent onset in an older child it may be due to a cranial nerve palsy (usually the VIth). In older children squint may be intermittent, or apparent rather than real because of epicanthic folds (Fig. 3.6). If the axes of the eyes are parallel, the reflections of a distant light on the corneae should occupy identical positions on the two eyes. In cases of doubt, or to demonstrate a latent squint, the *cover test* should be used (Fig. 3.6). Each eye should be covered and uncovered a few times whilst the observer looks carefully for movement of either eye.

Whilst this is being done the examiner should note any abnormality of the eye, e.g. opacities of the lens (cataract) or cornea, abnormalities of pupil size or shape.

In testing the Vth cranial nerve (trigeminal) it may be wise to avoid the corneal reflex which is an unpleasant experience.

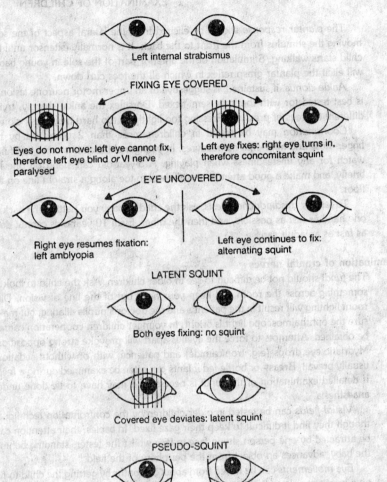

Left internal strabismus

FIXING EYE COVERED

Eyes do not move: left eye cannot fix, therefore left eye blind *or* VI nerve paralysed

Left eye fixes: right eye turns in, therefore concomitant squint

EYE UNCOVERED

Right eye resumes fixation: left amblyopia

Left eye continues to fix: alternating squint

LATENT SQUINT

Both eyes fixing: no squint

Covered eye deviates: latent squint

PSEUDO-SQUINT

Epicanthic folds: eyes appear to converge

Fig. 3.6. Examination of eyes for strabismus.

Cranial nerves VII–XII are tested as in adults. Facial weakness is usually obvious in an infant when he cries. The testing of vision and hearing are described on pp. 45 and 46.

Examination of the abdomen and perineum

Examination of the abdomen in children needs patience, gentleness and a warm hand. An older child will normally be happy to lie on a couch or bed (and will be happier with one pillow than with none), but a baby may be best examined on his mother's knee. An apprehensive toddler may also be best examined on her knee, or standing up beside her. The upright posture is maintained by the paravertebral muscles so the abdominal wall is relaxed.

Inspection is chiefly useful for detecting abdominal distension, visible peristalsis or hernia. Distension can be difficult to assess because of the very great normal variation. Fat babies appear to have bigger tummies than thin, muscular babies. Toddlers are normally rather pot-bellied in comparison with older children, and coloured children in comparison with white. The mother will usually be able to say whether the abdomen is swollen. If distension is caused by an intra-abdominal mass, its outline may be visible.

For *palpation* of the abdomen, it is helpful for the doctor to get down to the same level as the child by sitting or kneeling, unless the child is on a high bed or couch. This not only makes palpation more satisfactory, it makes conversation easier and the apprehensive child is saved from being towered over. If the abdominal muscles are tense, make small talk. An instruction to 'Relax!' tends to have the opposite effect. As with older patients, palpation should at first be very gentle, especially if some painful condition is suspected. The right side of the abdomen is sometimes more easily felt from the left side of the patient, either by going round the other side of the cot or by turning the child head to toes. Thus, the liver and the right kidney may be more easily felt. In suspected pyloric stenosis, examination must always be from the left side of the infant.

The liver is normally palpable in infants and toddlers. In babies, the edge is usually about 2 cm below the costal margin. A palpable spleen tip is not necessarily abnormal. The kidneys can usually be felt, the right more easily than the left, if the abdomen is reasonably thin and well relaxed. Faecal masses are commonly felt in the line of the colon. Small bowel peristalsis may be visible if the abdominal wall is very thin, as in small preterm babies and children with wasting diseases.

The main uses of *percussion* are to determine whether bowel overlies a palpable mass (an enlarged liver or spleen is dull: an enlarged kidney, unless massive, is resonant), and to detect ascites. Shifting dullness is a more useful sign than fluid thrill for detecting ascites.

Auscultation of the abdomen will reveal excessive bowel sounds if there is intestinal hurry (e.g. gastroenteritis) and in the early stages of intestinal obstruction. Abdominal silence (listen for several minutes) indicates bowel standstill, as in paralytic ileus.

Rectal examination is rarely omitted by surgeons and often forgotten by physicians. It may be disturbing to young or nervous children, and the decision whether or not to make a rectal examination depends upon what is likely to be learned from it. The doctor is unlikely to detect localized tenderness if the child is crying before he starts. The little finger should be used for rectal examination in infants, the index finger in older children.

Examination of a stool, which should be as fresh as possible, is often informative. The colour, consistency and smell are noted and the presence of blood or mucus.

The *testes* may be examined with the boy standing or lying. Far and away the most common problem is to distinguish between incompletely descended and retractile testes. The boy, and the doctor's hands, must be warm. A testis palpable in the groin can usually be 'milked' down into the scrotum. Testicular size can be assessed by comparison with a graded series of wooden ovoids of known volume (orchidometer).

The *prepuce* may be non-retractile until the boy is 3–4 years old because of normal adhesions between it and the glans. Thereafter gentle traction should be sufficient to retract it.

The *vaginal* and *urethral orifices* may need to be examined if there is a history of perineal irritation or discharge. Good illumination is essential: it is most easily performed with the child supine, the hips flexed and abducted. If vaginal examination is necessary, it is usually done under light, general anaesthesia (see also p. 202).

Urine examination (see p. 190 for details)

Examination of the urine is especially important in children. Infections are common and the symptoms may be non-specific. With a simple microscope, an acute urine infection can be diagnosed in 5 minutes. A laboratory report gives useful additional information but takes a day or two to complete.

Examination of the upper respiratory tract

This is an important part of the general examination of any child, especially an ill child. It is difficult in babies, and young children may dislike having their ears

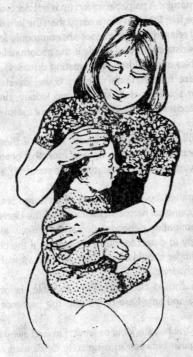

Fig. 3.7. Mother holding child ready for examination of ears. One hand presses the child's head securely to her chest, the other controls the child's outer arm, and presses inwards, so trapping the inner arm also.

examined. Practice makes perfect. The infant is held by the mother as shown in Fig. 3.7, her hands ensuring that the child's head is secure, so that the speculum cannot accidentally damage the meatus. The pinna is drawn gently upwards and backwards to allow a clear view of the ear drum. If wax obscures the view it must be gently removed with a wax hook or cotton wool on an orange stick. If the wax is very hard, softening ear drops may be needed first.

The nose should also be examined with the auriscope, noting the colour of the mucosa, the presence of oedema and secretions.

The mouth must be examined thoroughly, noting the state of the gums, teeth, tongue and buccal mucosa as well as the back of the throat. Older children will on request say 'Ah' and reveal the posterior pharynx. For younger children a good view is sometimes obtained by asking the child to put out his tongue. A wooden tongue depressor is well tolerated by most children provided it is used gently and is not placed so far back as to cause gagging. It is difficult to get a good view of the throat in babies. Never use force to view the throat of a young child with stridor: it may precipitate fatal respiratory obstruction

If the teeth look healthy, use the opportunity to congratulate the child. If there are problems of dental caries, misaligned teeth or malocclusion of the jaws, explain the need for early dental help.

Examination of the chest and lungs

Before laying a hand or a stethoscope on the child's chest, *look* at it and *listen* to his breathing. Inspection gives you information about the chest shape and the way it moves. Abnormalities of shape include the following:

1 *Hyperinflation* (usually called a barrel-shaped chest, which is inaccurate and offensive) caused by chronic or recurrent difficulty with expiration as in bad asthma.

2 *Pectus carinatum* (often called pigeon-chest, which is equally inaccurate and offensive) in which the sternum is displaced forwards relative to the anterior rib ends (Fig. 3.8).

3 *Pectus excavatum* results from a short central tendon of the diaphragm which tethers the lower end of the sternum, resulting in an epigastric saucer which may be quite deep.

4 *Harrison's sulcus* is caused by indrawing of the lower ribs at the line of attachment of the diaphragm. Originally described as a feature of rickets (in which the ribs are soft), it is now seen chiefly in severe asthma (in which the diaphragm may have to work overtime).

Abnormalities of chest movement include the following:

1 *Abnormalities of respiratory pattern.* The respiratory rate rises much more readily than in adults and reflects the severity of the disorder. It must be timed accurately: in infants, who often have irregular breathing, it should be timed over a full minute before the baby is disturbed or undressed. (It is meaningless to time a crying infant's respiration.) The respiratory rate in the neonatal period is 30–40/minute. By the age of 2 months the rate is under 30/minute.

Deep, sighing (acidotic) breathing is seen in diabetic precoma and in salicylate poisoning. Intermittent respiratory rhythm (periodic breathing) may be seen in neurological or terminal illness.

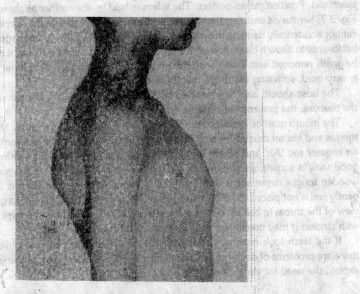

Fig. 3.8. Pectus carinatum. The boy also has a thoracic kyphosis which further exaggerates the anterior–posterior diameter of the chest.

2 *Asymmetry of chest movement*, best observed from the foot of the bed, is a helpful sign. The intrathoracic pathology is on (or worse on) the side that moves less well.

3 *Recession* of the intercostal spaces, epigastrium and suprasternal notch may occur during inspiration and means there is obstruction of the flow of air into the lungs.

Normal, quiet breathing is almost inaudible. *Wheeze* is a predominantly expiratory sound, characteristic of asthma at any age and of lower respiratory infections in young children. *Stridor* is a predominantly inspiratory sound indicative of airways obstruction in or near the larynx. Pharyngeal obstruction causes a similar but lower-pitch sound (stertor).

Cough in children most often arises in the upper respiratory tract and is rarely productive and purulent except in cystic fibrosis. Cough due to nasal or sinus catarrh is usually worst soon after going to bed and first thing in the morning. If due to throat infection it is a hard, dry, 'tickling' cough. If arising in the larynx it is croupy and sounds like a seal barking. If there is lung disease the cough may be moist and is often described as chesty. A paroxysmal cough, worse at night and on exertion, may be whooping cough without the whoop, but asthmatics are also inclined to cough under the same circumstances.

Tactile vocal fremitus is of little use in young children. Percussion should be done lightly, especially in babies. A thumping finger is more uncomfortable and less informative. Liver dullness starts at a higher level in young children than in adults and must not be mistaken for intrathoracic pathology.

For auscultation, use a stethoscope appropriate to the child's size. An adult-size diaphragm placed on a newborn baby will pick up heart, breath and bowel sounds all at once! Compare the volume of sound (often called air entry) at similar points on the two sides. The breath sounds in children are more bronchial and less vesicular than adult bronchovesicular breathing. They may be frankly bronchial, especially on the right, just lateral to the upper thoracic spine, being directly transmitted from the main bronchi.

Fine crepitations may only be audible on deep inspiration. A young child who cannot take a deep breath may be able to blow, and will then take a deep breath. Coarse crepitations may be sounds transmitted from the throat or upper airways. If he will cough, these sounds disappear.

Finger clubbing in children is rarely due to pulmonary disease except in cystic fibrosis.

Examination of the cardiovascular system

Inspection provides the most information, particularly in infants. Look at the chest. An enlarged right ventricle pushes the sternum forward. Look for increased respiratory rate (tachypnoea) and difficulty in breathing (dyspnoea), when the accessory muscles of respiration are used causing intercostal and subcostal recession, flaring of the alae nasi and recession in the suprasternal notch. These signs may result from heart or lung disease. Look for excessive sweating (an early sign of heart failure). Watch the baby feeding; he sucks well at first but then has to stop for a rest. The time taken for a feed is prolonged and insufficient feed is taken. The heart rate can be counted by watching the pulsation of the anterior fontanelle, but it is often difficult to study the neck veins in small children. Observation of the weight chart is important—a baby who is feeding poorly but gaining weight satisfactorily may be developing heart failure and accumulating fluid.

Cyanosis may be evident at rest or only on exertion, which for the infant means crying. In toddlers and older children minor degrees of arterial desaturation may show as a dark flush on the cheeks, a deceptive appearance suggesting rosy health. Cyanosis due to congenital heart disease increases on exertion and is usually associated with clubbing of the fingers and toes. Clubbing is not apparent until after 6 months of age and takes the same period to resolve after successful surgery.

Palpation

Feel the pulses in the arms and legs. The baby is less disturbed when the dorsalis pedis and tibial pulses are felt rather than the femorals. Variation in heart rate is often obvious, the rate increasing with inspiration and decreasing with expiration (sinus arrhythmia) (Table 3.3). Palpation over the heart to the left of the sternum demonstrates the activity of the right ventricle: there a heave indicates a high right ventricular pressure. The apex beat is usually just outside the nipple line in the 4th or 5th intercostal space; it gives information about the activity and volume of the left ventricle—when the heart is enlarged the apex is displaced towards the axilla. Feel for thrills and locate them accurately: the maximum site of a thrill is helpful in diagnosis. Remember that thrills may be felt in the neck: if

Table 3.3. Normal heart rates.

Age	Heart rate	
	Sleeping	Active
Fetus	120–160	
0–6 months	120	Up to 180
3 years	95	120
5 years	90	115
10 years	80	100
15 years	75	100

they occur in the neck alone the diagnosis is likely to be aortic stenosis. Feel for enlargement of the liver: it can often be seen distending the upper part of the abdomen and is dull to percussion.

Auscultation

The heart sounds are easier to hear in children than in adults. Splitting of the second sound is more obvious: it is wider in inspiration and narrows in expiration. A third sound is often heard at the cardiac apex and may mimic a diastolic murmur. Heart defects do not always cause heart murmurs, particularly in the newborn infant, but when murmurs are present the maximal site of the murmur is very helpful in diagnosis.

Blood pressure

The most important factor in recording the blood pressure is to use a cuff of the correct size. A variety of cuffs should always be available:

1   Width—this should cover two-thirds of the distance between the tips of the shoulder and elbow. It is best to apply a cuff as wide as possible: too small a cuff yields a false high blood pressure.

2   Length—the bladder should completely encircle the arm. Recordings of the blood pressure can be made by palpation (systolic), auscultation or using the flush method. In the flush method, the cuff is applied in the usual way and then, after wrapping a crêpe bandage firmly round the hand and forearm, the cuff is inflated above the expected systolic pressure and the bandage removed. The skin will be blanched. The sphygmomanometer pressure is then slowly lowered 5 mmHg at a time and the skin observed. A reading is made when the skin shows a pink flush. This pressure represents a point a little below the true systolic pressure. The same technique can be used to measure blood pressure in the legs, placing the cuff round the calf and the bandage round the foot.

Machines that use the oscillometric principle are now available and give accurate systolic and diastolic pressures as well as mean arterial pressure.

On the second day of life the mean systolic pressure is 70 mmHg, rising gradually over the next 6 weeks to a level of 93 mmHg. Thereafter the pressure remains remarkably level at 95 mmHg until 2 years of age. This level is maintained until the age of 6 years, after which it begins to rise very gradually, reaching levels of 125 mmHg by 16 years of age.

Examination of bones and joints

Fractures and bone infections are common in childhood and will cause local pain, tenderness and sometimes swelling. Joint disease is not so common, but arthritis and synovitis do occur. Each joint must be examined carefully:

1 *Inspection.* Is there swelling or deformity of the joint? Does the overlying skin look red? Compare the two sides. Is there wasting of adjacent muscles? If in doubt, measure. If any joint is painful, ask the child to show you how far it will move without pain before you touch it.

2 *Palpation.* Does the skin feel hot? Is there tenderness? Is there fluid in the joint? Is there crepitus when the joint moves? Put the joint through the full range of movement in every direction, watching the child's face to be sure you do not hurt him. Compare the two sides.

3 *Measurement.* Comparison of muscle bulk can be made by measuring the greatest circumference of the calves, upper arm or forearm muscles. Thighs should be measured about their middle, marking the same distance above the patella on the two sides. Leg lengths are measured with the legs in line with the trunk, from either the anterior superior iliac spine (which is not a very precise point) or the umbilicus to the medial malleolus at the ankle, taking the tape medial to the patella.

Joint movements

The *hip* movements are internal and external rotation, adduction, abduction in extension, abduction in flexion, flexion and (with the child prone) extension. Hip disease may be associated with buttock wasting and/or leg shortening. The method of testing for congenital dislocation of the hip is described on p. 178.

The *knee* normally extends beyond 180° and flexes until the heel touches the buttock. Knee disease is often associated with quadriceps wasting.

The *spine* (including the neck) should be examined for abnormal curvature and for mobility (forward and lateral flexion, extension, rotation).

The *shoulder* can be tested by asking the child to put his arms straight up in the air, then his hands behind his neck with elbows well back, then his hands behind his back.

The *wrist* normally flexes and extends through 180°.

DEVELOPMENTAL ASSESSMENT

This is an important part of any health check in young children and in children presenting with developmental delay (late walking, late talking). It is not the first priority in an acutely ill child. The main purposes of developmental assessment are:

1 To detect early any significant departure from the wide range of normal so that any necessary help (advice, spectacles, hearing aid) can be provided early.

2 In the great majority of children, to provide reassurance to parents that all is going well.

Developmental tests are sometimes thought of as pass/fail tests, competitive tests or prognostic tests. All three are wrong.2nd half of figure 3.9

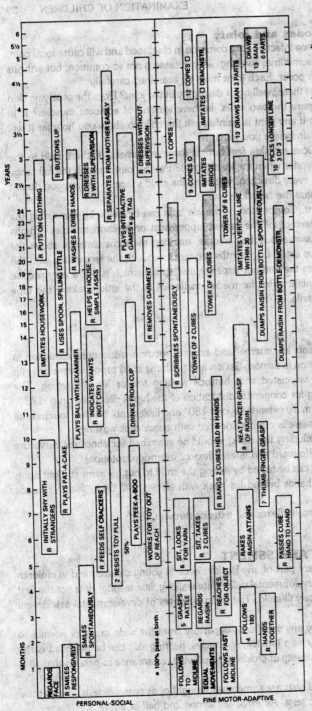

Fig. 3.9. Denver Developmental Screening Charts. Each box relates to a different skill. Those preceded by the letter 'R' mean that the tester relies on the report of the child's parent. Other skills are observed by the tester (the numbers on the left of some boxes refer to the footnotes 1–28). Twenty five percent of children pass the test by the age signified by the left edge of the box and 90% by the right edge. The shaded area signifies the 75–90th centile, and the vertical line on top of the box the 50th centile.

(1) Get child to smile—do not touch him. (2) Pull toy away from child when playing—pass if he resists. (3) Child need not tie shoes or do up back buttons. (4) Move yarn in an arc, 6″ above child's face. Pass if eyes follow 90° to midline. (5) Pass if child grasps rattle touched to back or tips of fingers. (6) Pass if child looks where yarn goes (tester should drop yarn quickly without arm movement). (7) Pass if child picks up raisin with any part of thumb and finger. (8) Pass if child picks up raisin with end of thumb and index finger. (9) Get child to copy circle—pass any enclosed form, fail continuous spiral. (10) Get child to indicate the longer line (not bigger). Repeat with paper turned upsidedown (3/3 or 5/6). (11) Get child to copy cross—pass any crossing lines. (12) Get child to copy square—demonstrate if he fails. Do not name forms in 9, 11 and 12. Do not demonstrate 9 and 11.

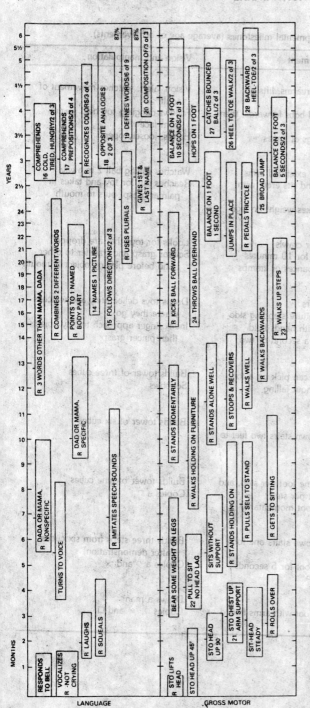

Footnotes contd.

(13) When scoring, each pair counts as one part. (14) Get child to name animal picture (no credit for sounds only). (15) Tell child 'give Mummy block'; 'put block on table/floor'—pass 2 of 3. (16) Ask child 'what do you do when cold/hungry/tired?'—pass 2 of 3. (17) Tell child to put block on table, under table, etc. do not help with signs. (18) Ask child 'if fire is hot, ice is -?' 'horse is big, mouse is -?' etc. Pass 2 or 3. (19) Ask child 'what is ball/lake/desk/hedge, etc.?' 'Pass if defined by use, shape or category.—Pass 6 of 9. (20) Ask child 'what is spoon/shoe/door made of?'—Pass 3 of 3. (21) Child can lift chest with support of arms or hands when on stomach. (22) Grasp hands and pull to sitting when child is on back—pass if head does not hang back. (23) Child climbs steps using wall or rail (not crawling). (24) Child throws ball overhand to within 3" of tester's arm reach. (25) Child jumps 8½" from standing. (26) Child walks forwards for 4 consecutive steps, heel within 1" of toe. Pass 2 of 3 trials (can demonstrate). (27) Bounce ball to child 3' away, pass if he catches with hands not arms, 2 of 3 trials. (28) Child walks backwards (toe within 1" of toe for 4 steps)—pass 2 of 3 trials (may demonstrate).

Table 3.4 Developmental milestones (average age of achievements).

Posture and movement	Vision and manipulation
3 months Prone: rests on forearms, lifts up head and chest Pulled to sit: head bobs forwards, then held erect Held standing: sags at knees	Vision: alert, watches movement of adult Follows dangling toy held 15 cm from face Hands: loosely open
6 months Prone: lifts up on extended arms Pulls self to sit, and sits erect with support Held standing: takes weight on legs	Watches rolling ball 2 m away Reaches out for toy and takes in palmar grasp, puts to mouth
9 months Prone: wriggles or crawls Sits unsupported for 10 minutes Held standing: bounces or stamps	Looks for toys that are dropped Scissor grasp and transfer to other hand before placing object in mouth
1 year Crawls on all fours Walks round furniture stepping side-ways. Walks with hands held Stands alone for a second or two	Drops toys deliberately and watches where they go Index finger approach to tiny objects, then pincer grasp
1½ years Walks alone and can pick up a toy from floor without falling	Builds tower of three cubes Scribbles
2 years Runs Walks up and down stairs two feet to a step	Builds tower of six cubes
3 years Walks upstairs one foot per step, and down two feet per step Stands on one foot momentarily	Builds tower of nine cubes Copies a ○
4 years Walks up and down stairs one foot per step Stands on one foot for 5 seconds	Builds three steps from six cubes (after demonstration) Copies a ○ and ×
5 years Skips. Hops Stands on one foot with arms folded for 5 seconds	Draws a man Copies ○, × and □

Table 3.4. (continued)

Hearing and speech	Social behaviour
Quietens to interesting sounds Chuckles and coos when pleased	Shows pleasure appropriately

Localizes soft sounds 45 cm
   (18 inches) lateral to either ear
Makes double syllable sounds and
   tuneful noises
	Alert, interested
	Still friendly with strangers

Brisk localization of soft sounds
   1 m (3 feet) lateral to either ear
Babbles tunefully
	Distinguishes strangers and shows
	   apprehension
	Chews solids

Understands simple commands Babbles incessantly	Cooperates with dressing, e.g. holding up arms Waves bye-bye
Uses several words, sound labels	Drinks from cup using two hands Demands constant mothering
Joins words together in simple • phrases, as sound ideas	Uses spoon Indicates toilet needs, dry by day Play imitates adult activities
Speaks in sentences Gives full name	Eats with spoon and fork Can undress with assistance Dry by night

Talks a lot
Speech contains many infantile
   substitutions
	Dresses and undresses with
	   assistance

Fluent speech with few infantile substitutions	Dresses and undresses alone Washes and dries face and hands

1 The tests to be described are essentially screening tests, designed to identify children who need detailed, expert examination of one or more developmental fields (e.g. hearing).

2 The child who walks earlier than his peers will not necessarily prove to be more intelligent.

3 Global delay (that is, delay in all fields) is certainly worrying, but late motor development is of less certain significance than late social development. The less marked the delay and the younger the child, the more cautious is the wise doctor in predicting the future.

Developmental skills fall into four categories:

1 Posture and movement.
2 Vision and manipulation (hand/eye coordination).
3 Hearing and speech.
4 Social behaviour.

There are two parts to a developmental assessment, the history presented by the mother and the doctor's own observations. Be sure the medical record keeps them separate. The history is usually reliable and augments the clinical examination, but the parents of retarded or handicapped children may exaggerate their abilities or misinterpret, for example, involuntary movements as efforts to achieve something.

1 *The history.* The mother should be encouraged to give a careful account of the child's present skills, ensuring that each of the four main categories is covered. If there are older siblings, it is helpful to enquire how the child's skills compare with those of the siblings at that age. Enquire about school performance if the child is at school for he is unlikely to have a significant developmental problem if he is coping well in a normal class of children of similar age. Try to obtain information about the dates of the early milestones. Some mothers recall them well, others not at all. If an experienced mother says 'he was very quick' it may not be necessary to obtain exact detail of past achievements.

2 *Play with the child*—in the presence of the mother so as to encourage the child to show certain skills.

Try to define the limit of achievement by noting both the skills the child *has* and those he has *not*. The Denver Developmental Screening Test charts (Fig. 3.9) are useful for recording information, and for practising developmental assessment. The following simple tests require equipment that is available in any surgery or clinic, and require no special expertise on the part of the examiner. The ages given are the *average* ages at which the skill is seen. Refer also to Table 3.4.

1 Posture and movement

Body control is acquired from the top downwards:

Head on trunk—the newborn baby held upright can balance his head briefly. Laid on his back and pulled up by arms or shoulders, there is complete head lag. By 4 months the head comes up in line with the trunk. By 6 months the head comes up in advance of the trunk.

Trunk on pelvis—by 7 months a baby can sit briefly on a firm, flat surface, often using his arms for support. By 9 months he sits without arm support and can turn without falling.

Pelvis on legs—by 10 months he can pull himself up to stand and begins to cruise round the furniture. By 12–15 months he can walk unaided.

2 Vision and manipulation (hand–eye coordination)

1 Visual attention. At 8 weeks a baby observes with a convergent gaze a dangling toy or bright object held 23–30 cm (9–12 inches) from his face, and moves his head and neck in order to follow it. A true squint (as distinct from a pseudo-squint as seen with epicanthic folds) is always abnormal and requires referral to a specialist (see p. 103).

From 2 months a baby prefers to watch a face rather than anything else, but more detailed testing is possible with care and special equipment. The Stycar testing kit includes:

(a) A series of white balls of different sizes which are rolled across the floor in front of the baby. At 6–9 months a baby will watch a ball as small as 4 mm diameter at a distance of 3 m.

(b) Two sets of miniature dolls-house type toys and cutlery. The toddler has one set and points to the item which is the same as that held by the tester 3 m away.

(c) Letter matching cards which can be used at 3–6 years, even though the child has not yet learnt letters. The child points to one of the five letters on his card which is the same as a single letter held by the tester 3 m away.

2 Grasp. A wooden tongue depressor or spatula is held before the infant. At 6 months he approaches it with the ulnar border of the hand and then takes it in a clumsy palmar grasp. At 9 months he approaches it with the radial border and takes it in a scissor grasp between the sides of thumb and index finger before transferring it to the other hand and putting in in his mouth. At 12 months he approaches it with the index finger and picks it up precisely between the ends of the thumb and index finger in a pincer grasp (Fig. 3.10).

3 Copying. A child will copy with a pencil the following shapes:

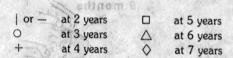

| or —   at 2 years   □   at 5 years
○   at 3 years   △   at 6 years
+   at 4 years   ◇   at 7 years

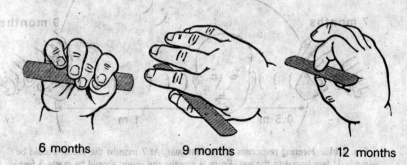

6 months   9 months   12 months

Fig. 3.10. Palmar grasp at 6 months, scissor grasp at 9 months and pincer grasp at 12 months.

Building and copying with blocks. Small wooden 2.5 cm (1-inch) cubes are best. The child will copy:

at 1½ years, a tower of 3 cubes   at 3, a 'bridge'

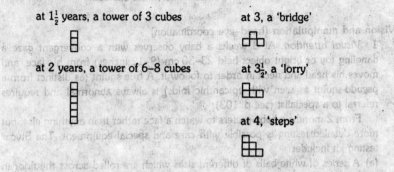

at 2 years, a tower of 6–8 cubes   at 3½, a 'lorry'

at 4, 'steps'

3 Hearing and speech

Localization of sounds. The baby is sat on mother's knee facing another adult about 3 m (10 feet) away whose function is to keep the baby's visual attention straight ahead (but without being so fascinating that the baby ignores the test sounds).

A variety of soft sounds are made lateral to either ear and out of the line of vision. Rustling soft tissue or toilet paper provides a high-frequency sound; a spoon gently scraped round a cup, or a high-pitched rattle are other suitable sounds. Provided the baby has reasonable hearing he will turn to locate the source. At 7 months the baby turns to sounds 0.5 m (1½ feet) from either ear. At 9 months he turns promptly to sounds 1 m (3 feet) away, even if they are situated diagonally (Fig. 3.11). The optimal age at which to test an infant's hearing is 7 months.

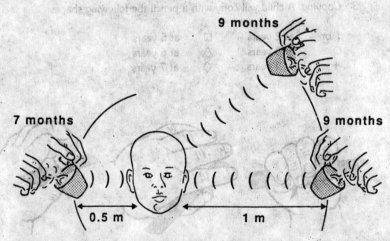

Fig. 3.11. Hearing responses in the first year. At 7 months the sound should be made 1½ feet lateral to the ear. From 9 months the sound should be made 3 feet lateral to the ear.

These distraction tests are for screening only. An infant who does not respond normally without good cause (e.g. coryza) must be referred promptly for detailed assessment (see p. 104).

Speech. At 9 months there is varied and tuneful babbling. From 1 year single word *labels* are used for familiar objects and people—'Mum'. 'Dog'. He will look towards a named object, e.g. 'Where's the ball?' At 2 years words are joined to convey *ideas*—'Dadad gone' and will follow simple instructions, e.g. 'Put the spoon in the cup'. At 3, sentences are used to describe present and past happenings. Throughout this period the child's understanding of language is far ahead of his ability to utter it.

4 Social behaviour

Smiling. In response to mother's face smiling is seen at 4–8 weeks.

Reacting to strangers. Up to 9 months most babies will be happily handled by anyone; from 9 months they begin to cry or fret if handled by a stranger.

Feeding. At 9 months, lumpy food is properly chewed. At 18 months, the child cooperates with feeding, and drinks from an ordinary cup using two hands. At 3 years, he can feed himself efficiently with a spoon and fork.

Limitations of developmental assessment

Technique

As with any examination the expert will always get the most reliable information, but anyone who is willing to listen to the mother and observe the child can get some useful information about each of the four main fields of development. If the mother's account differs greatly from what is observed, it may be that the child is having an 'off day', in which case observing on another occasion will be more reliable.

Range of normal

The age at which a normal child achieves a particular physical or developmental goal is extremely variable; 50% of children can walk 10 steps unaided at 13 months, but a few can do this at 8 months, and others not until 18 months. It is kinder to talk to parents of the 'usual' age for developing a skill rather than the 'normal', since abnormal implies a fault. Quite commonly one field of activity appears delayed in a normal child, but it is rare for all four fields of development to be delayed if the child is normal.

Milestones are stepping stones

Parents tend to think of certain developmental skills as essential milestones. It is truer to regard them as stepping stones. In general one cannot reach a particular stepping stone without using the previous ones—and a child does not run until he can walk or walk until he can stand. But different people may use different stepping stones, and occasionally miss one out. Most children crawl before they stand, but some shuffle on their bottoms, never crawl, yet stand and walk normally in the end. Bottom shuffling is a typical example of the sort of variation in development that can cause parents much unnecessary worry, particularly as bottom shufflers tend to walk later than other children.

Using stepping stones we may go in sudden bounds rather than at an even rate—children often develop that way, appearing static for a few weeks then suddenly mastering a new skill. If the next stepping stone is a particularly hard one, all the child's energy may appear to be devoted to just one of the four fields of development, whilst the other three seem static; posture and movement skills may advance rapidly about the age of 1 year as walking is mastered, whilst hearing and speech development appear static.

The first 6 months

This is the most difficult time to assess the baby, because it is not until about 6 months that many of the easier developmental tests can be used. Therefore, developmental testing before the age of 6 months is less reliable than at any other time.

FURTHER READING

Buckler JMH. A Reference Manual of Growth and Development. Blackwell Scientific Publications.

Denver Developmental Screening Test, 1967. J. Paediatrics, 71, 185. (The charts are available from the Test Agency, Counswood House, North Dean, High Wycombe, Buckinghamshire.)

Egan D, Illingworth RS and MacKeith RC Development Screening 0–5 Yrs. Clinics in Developmental Medicine 30. Heinemann.

Falkner F and Tanner JM (eds). Human Growth, Baillière Tindall.

Illingworth RS. The Development of the Infant and Young Child. Churchill Livingstone.

Tanner JM. Foetus into Man. Castlemead Publications.

Chapter 4
The Unborn Baby

Traditionally, paediatricians have been concerned with children from the moment of their birth while obstetricians have expressed their concern for the fetus indirectly through their care of the mother. This approach has been quietly revolutionized over the past 25 years as a result of three separate phenomena:

1 Thalidomide created an awareness that the embryo and fetus are profoundly affected by the maternal environment.

2 Amniocentesis, ultrasound scanning, fetal blood sampling and chorion villus biopsy rendered the fetus accessible to examination and investigation.

3 Legislation regarding the termination of pregnancy and, more recently, *in vitro* fertilization, has forced the entire community to recognize the fetus as a human being and to consider, if not to solve, some difficult moral problems.

Before considering the health of the unborn baby it is important to appreciate the relationship between contraception and child health. This may sound paradoxical, but high birth rates and high child mortality tend to go hand in hand. In developing countries, large families are usual in the hope that a few will survive to adult life. Medical care reduces mortality from disease, but unless family size is reduced *pari passu*, the children may die from starvation instead. The theory is simple: its translation into practice depends upon the availability of safe, effective, cheap contraception coupled with education of the community to accept it.

In vitro fertilization

Whilst contraception has been with us for a very long time, methods of helping infertile couples to have babies (other than by adoption) have been revolutionized by the technique of *in vitro* fertilization ('test-tube babies'). This permits the separation of functions previously regarded as more or less inseparable:

1 The provision of one or more ova.

2 The provision of sperm.

3 The place of fertilization.

4 The uterus in which the fetus develops.

5 The adult(s) responsible for rearing the child.

Hence the ovum could come from Ms A, be fertilized in the laboratory by sperm from Mr B, be implanted in the uterus of Ms C and be reared by Mr and Ms D. Doctors need to be aware of the likely effects on the child of the more bizarre variations on this theme. The Warnock Report suggested guidelines for legislation.

Pre-pregnancy care

Conventional antenatal care begins when a pregnant woman first presents herself to a doctor or midwife. This provides an opportunity to ensure that in due course labour takes place in the safest place; at the safest time and in the safest hands. It is, however, too late to affect some of the important influences on the early development of the embryo and fetus. It is for this reason that pre-pregnancy (pre-conception) clinics are gradually beginning to gain ground. The following are among the matters deserving consideration:

1   The transition from contraception to pregnancy. It is generally advised that oral contraceptives should be stopped at least 3 months before conceiving.

2   The physical and emotional health of both partners. Not only should they be well and ready for parenthood, but hereditary conditions which might affect the child can be discussed.

3   A review of personal habits relating to eating, drinking, smoking and drug-taking, including prescribed drugs. The importance of good nutrition in pregnancy has been rediscovered.

Alcohol in excess (and nobody is quite sure how much that is) can interfere with normal development, and both alcohol and smoking can interfere with growth in the unborn baby. The correction of bad habits in the course of pregnancy may suffice to allow normal growth to be resumed, but congenital deformities cannot be undone. Many drugs have some teratogenic potential and all but the most essential should be stopped before pregnancy. Most drugs given to a pregnant women reach the unborn baby.

4   Immunity to rubella (German measles) can be checked by a blood test, and susceptible women immunized before becoming pregnant.

Congenital malformations

About 2% of all babies are born with serious congenital defects, sufficient to threaten life, to cause permanent handicap, or to require surgical correction. Malformations therefore form a major cause of perinatal and infant death, and constitute one of the greatest problems in paediatrics. Defects of the central nervous system and heart account for more than half the total. Most of the common defects are described in the relevant chapters: here some general principles will be considered.

Distressingly little is known of the causes of congenital abnormalities. Single-gene defects and chromosome anomalies account for 10–20% of the total. A small number are attributable to intrauterine infections (e.g. cytomegalovirus, rubella), fewer to teratogenic drugs and even fewer to ionizing radiation. The causes of most common defects remain unknown, although some aetiological factors are known. For example, some defects are more common in certain ethnic groups, socioeconomic groups, or at some maternal ages and parities than others. It is believed that most non-genetic defects arise from the simultaneous action of many adverse factors upon a susceptible embryo.

The incidence of serious defects and chromosomal anomalies amongst early spontaneous abortuses is very high. Nature has devised a fairly efficient system for terminating at the first possible moment pregnancies that are doomed to failure. It can be shown, for example, that at least 90% of embryos/fetuses with trisomy 21, and a much higher proportion of embryos with sex chromosome anomalies, are aborted. Live-born, malformed infants therefore represent the small minority for which this mechanism has failed.

Prenatal diagnosis

Prenatal diagnosis can be helpful because:

1 It may influence the management of pregnancy and delivery.
2 Termination of pregnancy may need to be considered.
3 There are increasing opportunities for intrauterine treatment.

The variety of techniques for monitoring the growth and development of the fetus is expanding all the time.

1 *Ultrasonography* has become part of routine antenatal care. It is used principally to monitor growth and to determine gestational age, but it will inevitably detect many structural defects of the fetus including missing structures (anencephaly), enlarged organs (polycystic kidneys), soft-tissue swellings (encephalocele) and bodily disporportion (skeletal dysplasias).

2 *Amniocentesis* involves the withdrawal of a sample of amniotic fluid, usually around the 16th week of pregnancy. A wide variety of tests can be carried out on cells, which are of fetal origin, and on the supernatant fluid. Alphafetoprotein (AFP) is raised with open neural-tube defects, exomphalos and some other defects. Acetylcholinesterase is more specific to neural defects. Cells can be cultured for karyotyping or genetic tests. A wide range of metabolic disorders can be diagnosed prenatally. Amniocentesis carries a small risk of causing miscarriage and is therefore used selectively for mothers at raised risk of having an abnormal fetus, either because of a family history of genetic disorder or, in the case of Down's syndrome, because of advanced parental age.

3 *Serum AFP screening* is not a diagnostic procedure but a risk-free means of identifying a subgroup of pregnant women who may have raised amniotic fluid AFP. Many antenatal clinics offer the screening test to all patients.

4 *Fetoscopy* and fetal blood sampling are not widely available, are not without risk, and are appropriate for a strictly limited number of women. Fetoscopy will reveal some defects not recognizable with an ultrasound scan. Fetal blood samples may be taken for tests.

5 *Chorion villus biopsy* is carried out at about 10 weeks of pregnancy and can provide material for chemical and genetic analysis. This technique carries a small risk of miscarriage.

Later in pregnancy, an excess or deficiency of amniotic fluid (polyhydramnios:oligohydramnios) may be a sign of fetal abnormality. A fetus that cannot swallow (oesophageal atresia, anencephaly) is often associated with polyhydramnios; a fetus that cannot urinate (renal agenesis) with oligohydramnios.

Growth and development of the embryo and fetus

In early pregnancy the embryological timetable is important in relation to possible teratogenic hazards—infective, chemical or physical agents that may cause birth defects. In the middle trimester of pregnancy, growth, as estimated from uterine size and ultrasound measurement of the fetal skull, is an important indicator of fetal well-being, as it is of health after birth.

The major structural and functional developments in the embryo are summarized in Table 4.1.

The increase in size of the human from conception to birth is phenomenal. Increase in length is only 1 mm/week for the first 5 weeks but then accelerates to

Table 4.1. Embryological development of the fetus.

Days	Weeks	Crown-rump length (mm)	General body form and skeletal system	Nervous systems and sense organs	Cardiovascular and respiratory systems	Digestive system	Genitourinary system
0	0	0	Ovum Zygote Blastocyst Implantation				
	1						
10	2	1		Neural plate	Cardiogenic plate		
20	3	2	Somites	Optic vesicle Otocyst Ant. neuropore closes Post. neuropore closes	Heart tubes fuse 1st aortic arch	Fore and hindgut	Pronephros
	4	4	Anterior limb buds Posterior limb buds		Heart beating Lung primordia Septum primum Aortic arches	Liver bud	Mesonephros
30	5		Myotomes	Olfactory pits	Primary and lobar bronchi Septum secundum IV septum	Stomach primordium Dorsal pancreas	Metanephros Genital ridge
	6	10	Finger rays Cartilaginous models	Primordium of cerebellum Retinal pigment Pinnae forming	Ductus venosus Division of truncus	Ventral pancreas Spleen Umbilical hernia Division of cloaca	Primordium of gonad
	7	20	Primary ossification centres	Eyelids Semicircular canals	Septa complete Segmental bronchi	Haemopoiesis in liver	
50	8		Separate digits Palatal processes grow medially		Main blood vessels present	Rectum and bladder separated Lumen in gall bladder	Gonadal differentiation Müllerian primordium
60	9	30	Palatal fusion	Differentiation of cerebral cortex		Umbilical hernia	Uterus complete Gonad differentiated

1 mm/day and by 8 weeks to 1.5 mm/day. At this age the embryo weighs about 1 g. Subsequent weights average 14 g at 3 months, 105 g at 4 months, 310 g at 5 months, 640 g at 6 months (about the lower limit of viability), and thereafter a rate of weight gain rising from 100 to 250 g/week.

The growth of the fetus is traditionally assessed by estimation of uterine size, but more accurately by serial ultrasound scans. Functional development can be judged by a variety of techniques ranging from the mother's awareness of fetal movements to estimation of fetal lung maturity by measurements of lipids in amniotic fluid. It is primarily upon the developmental maturity of the lungs and brain that the survival of very small preterm babies depends (p. 66).

Chapter 5
The Newborn

Healthy transition from intrauterine to extrauterine life is a vital step in the development of an individual. To accomplish it, the fetus must escape the potentially damaging aspects of the birth process, conduct major physiological changes to adapt to a new environment, and subsequently, as a neonate, evade the environmental hazards such as hypothermia and infection, to which he is particularly susceptible. If he is compelled to make the transition before he is ready, if he has encountered adverse intrauterine influences such as hypoxia or malnutrition or if he is among the 2% of babies with a major congenital abnormality, then the intrapartum and early neonatal period are especially hazardous. There is a greater risk of dying on the first day of life than on any other day (except the last) and a significant proportion of the population is handicapped in some way or another by perinatal events. Since almost all of this mortality and morbidity is potentially preventable, the perinatal period offers a unique opportunity to practise effective medicine.

THE EFFECTS OF BIRTH ON THE FETUS

Normal physiology. The most dramatic physiological events related to birth are the switch from placenta to lung as the organ of gas exchange, and the change from fetal to adult circulation that this necessitates. The major phenomena involved in this transition are set out in Table 5.1.

The right and left sides of the heart are now connected in series rather than in parallel, and the conversion is completed by anatomical closure of the foramen ovale and the ductus arteriosus (see p. 135). Most fetuses conduct these events efficiently; a minority suffer potentially damaging asphyxia along the way.

Perinatal asphyxia

For reasons which are not fully understood the placenta oxygenates fetal blood to a Pao_2 of only about 4 kPa, which equates to the arterial Pao_2 of man at the summit of Mount Everest. Nevertheless, the oxygen requirements of the fetus are fully met thanks to adaptations such as the high cardiac output (200 ml/kg/min), high haemoglobin concentration (18 g/dl), and the left-shifted dissociation curve of fetal haemoglobin (HbF) which allows greater oxygen saturation of haemoglobin at a given Pao_2. The fetus sits on the steep part of the dissociation curve, however, so that only a small drop in Pao_2 will result in a large reduction in blood oxygen content. As a result, oxygenation around the time of birth is in a state of delicate balance which depends critically on many factors, the most important of which are shown in Table 5.2.

Note that hypoxia can interfere with the function of the respiratory centre, leading to apnoea after birth and a vicious circle of hypoxia.

54

Table 5.1. Normal physiological events at birth.

Phenomena	Effects
Stress of labour stimulates catecholamine and steriod responses in fetus	Prepares lung for air breathing by curtailing lung liquid secretion and stimulating surfactant release
Uterine contractions impede villous space blood flow	Deteriorating trend in fetal blood gas status
Compression of fetal thorax by birth canal	Expulsion of some lung liquid
Thorax recoils on leaving birth canal	Proximal airway fills with air
Blood gases deteriorate following clamping of the umbilical cord	Initiation of breathing
Bombardment by sensory stimuli, e.g. cold	Initiation of breathing
Air enters lungs and raises interstitial Po_2	Pulmonary vascular resistance falls, with resulting increases in pulmonary blood flow, arterial Po_2 and left atrial filling
Low resistance placental circulation stops	Systemic vascular resistance increases and venous return to right atrium falls
Pressure gradient between atria reverses	Foramen ovale closes functionally
Direction of ductal shunt reverses and ductus perfused with oxygen-rich blood	Ductus arteriosus closes

Table 5.2. Perinatal oxygen supply.

Requirements	Potential threats
Normal maternal Pao_2	Severe cardiorespiratory disease. Hypoxia during anaesthesia
Adequate uterine blood flow	Maternal hypotension due to hyperventilation or anaesthesia. Compression of abdominal aorta or inferior vena cava by uterus. Maternal vascular disease (e.g. pre-eclampsia, diabetes). Prolonged or obstructed labour
Healthy placenta	Placental infarction. Placental abruption. Intrauterine infection. Substantial post-maturity
Unobstructed umbilical cord blood flow	Cord compression by fetal parts. Cord prolapse. Torn or knotted cord
A normal fetal haemoglobin concentration	Rhesus haemolytic disease. Twin-to-twin transfusion
Functioning respiratory centre	Intrapartum hypoxia. Respiratory depressant drugs
Patent airway	Obstruction by meconium or blood. Choanal atresia
Healthy heart and lungs	Lung immaturity. Diaphragmatic hernia. Severe congenital heart disease

In view of the frequency of some of the threats in Table 5.2 it is not surprising that the fetus has evolved defences against acute hypoxia, which include redistribution of blood flow in favour of vital tissues, and a myocardium and nervous system better able to withstand anaerobic conditions than the equivalent adult organs. Only a small minority of fetuses suffer perinatal brain damage, although many more experience lesser degrees of hypoxia which call for prompt obstetric action and resuscitation at birth in order to prevent progression.

Hypoxia before birth should be suspected when there is evidence of fetal growth retardation, reduced blood flow in the umbilical or arcuate arteries (measured by Doppler ultrasound), abnormalities of the fetal heart beat, reduction in liquor volume, reduced fetal movements or meconium staining of the liquor. If necessary it can be confirmed by fetal blood sampling. At birth the presence of asphyxia is recognized by observation of respiratory activity and heart rate, muscle tone, skin colour and reflex activity. These may be evaluated by the Apgar scoring system as shown in Table 5.3.

A total score of 10 is possible for the healthiest of infants, whereas badly asphyxiated infants usually score 3 or less. When scored at 1 and 5 minutes after birth the Apgar score is a useful assessment of the condition of the newborn, but the need for resuscitation can rapidly be assessed on the basis of the heart rate and breathing activity.

Any baby who does not breathe within 30 seconds of birth, or who exhibits slow and irregular gasping requires help. In order to reduce the risk of hypothermia during resuscitation the baby should be quickly dried with a towel and placed on a resuscitation platform with a radiant heat source. First the mouth, and then the nose are cleared of secretions with a soft suction catheter. If the heart rate is 100 or more beats per minute, hypoxia is not far advanced and breathing can usually be started or improved by gentle cutaneous stimulation or by flicking the soles of the feet. If there is no response to these simple measures, or if the heart rate is below 100 beats per minute, especially if the baby is pale, limp and immobile, intermittent positive pressure ventilation is begun either by bag and mask or by an endotracheal tube (Fig. 5.1). If the mother has received opiate analgesia, naloxone hydrochloride, 200 microgrammes intramuscularly is given to counteract respiratory depression.

Infants who make a rapid recovery should be given to their mothers as soon as possible, and only the tiny minority of severely asphyxiated babies need be admitted to a special care baby unit for further care.

Table 5.3. Apgar score.

Sign	0	1	2
Heart rate	Absent	Below 100/min	100/min or higher
Respiratory effort	Nil	Slow, irregular	Regular, with cry
Muscle tone	Limp	Some tone in limbs	Active movements
Reflex irritability	Nil	Grimace only	Cry
Colour	Pallor or generalized cyanosis	Body pink, extremities blue	Pink all over

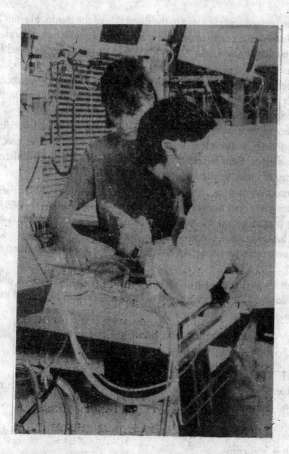

Fig. 5.1. Endotracheal intubation on the labour ward.

The prognosis in asphyxia bears a better relationship to the neurological state of the baby during the first week of life than to any assessment made immediately at or shortly after birth.

ROUTINE CARE OF THE NORMAL BABY

Vitamin K. Newborn babies have low levels of vitamin K and its dependent clotting factors, and some of them will bleed during the first few days of life, from the gastrointestinal tract, into the skin or mucous membranes, or at some other site. Most hospitals give 1 mg of vitamin K intramuscularly at birth. The only babies who nowadays suffer from 'haemorrhagic disease of the newborn' are those in whom the injection has been forgotten.

Umbilical cord. The two umbilical arteries are identified, as a single artery may be associated with congenital malformation. The cord is clamped about

1 cm from the skin surface and cut close to the distal side of the clamp. Most units use some form of antiseptic preparation on the cord stump until it has separated, which is usually by about one week. The cord should be carefully observed for signs of infection.

Labelling. There is a risk of mistaken identity and all newborn babies should have name bands attached to wrist and ankle in the delivery room and in the presence of the mother.

Bathing. Although it is tempting to wash the newborn clean of the debris picked up during birth, bathing carries a serious risk of cooling and can be deferred for a few days. Skin vernix is absorbed naturally. The umbilical cord should be kept dry in order to prevent infection.

Passage of meconium and urine. It is important to note the time of first passing meconium and urine. Sometimes this occurs at or soon after delivery, but both are usually passed within 12 hours of birth (although meconium passage may be delayed beyond this in some normal babies).

Delay in bowel or bladder function should prompt a search for underlying pathology.

Feeding. This topic is dealt with fully in Chapter 6. The first feed, of either breast milk or a formula, should be offered within 3–6 hours of birth, and there is much to be said for putting the baby to the breast shortly after birth.

EXAMINATION OF THE NEWBORN

All newborn babies should have a clinical examination within the first 24 hours of life, and a second check at about 1 week. The aims are to:

1 Detect
   (a) conditions that will benefit from early treatment, e.g. congenital dislocation of the hip, glaucoma:
   (b) conditions needing long-term supervision, e.g. congenital heart disease, club foot:
   (c) conditions that have genetic implications for future pregnancies, e.g. Down's syndrome:
   (d) signs of systemic illness:

2 Discuss parental anxieties, and to take a brief medical, genetic and social history, seeking information that may be relevant to the future health and development of the baby.

3 Provide advice on matters such as infant feeding, attendance at baby clinics, and immunization.

4 Note and advise on minor abnormalities about which parents may otherwise worry (see Table 5.4).

The following scheme of physical examination is in common use. It is not directed at diagnosing symptomatic illness, and it assumes that gross external abnormalities have been detected already. It is performed in the presence of the mother so that the doctor can explain what is being done.

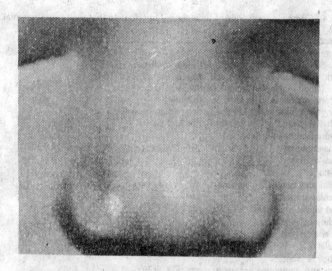

Fig. 5.2. Milia. Characteristically the small, raised, white spots are most prominent over the nose and upper cheeks.

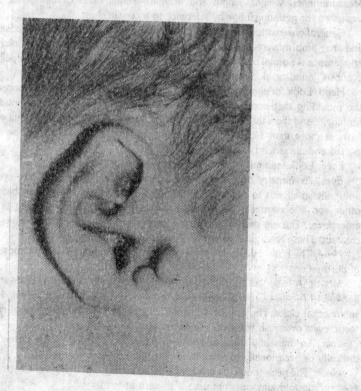

Fig. 5.3. Pre-auricular skin tags or 'accessory' auricles.

Table 5.4. Common conditions of little clinical importance that may cause parental anxiety.

Skin lesions:
1   strawberry naevi—which take a few days to appear (p. 184)
2   'stork' marks on the eyelids and nape of the neck (p. 184)
3   milia (small white skin lesions on the face) (Fig. 5.2)
4   urticaria neonatorum (a rash on the trunk)
5   'mongolian' blue spots (on the back in Asian babies)
6   epithelial 'pearls' in the mouth (gums and palate)
Subconjunctival haemorrhage
Cephalhaematoma
Positional talipes
Tongue-tie
Peripheral and traumatic cyanosis
Breast enlargement
Oral and vulval mucosal tags
Sacral dimple
Eyelid oedema
Hydrocele
Physiological jaundice
Skin tags and diminutive accessory digits (Fig. 5.3)

Suggested scheme for routine clinical examination

Measurements. Weight, length and occipito–frontal head circumference are evaluated for gestational age by reference to a centile chart.

General observation. Check that the infant exhibits the normal flexed posture and that limb movements are symmetrical. Ask yourself whether the infant's appearance is normal or whether there are dysmorphic features. Look for pallor, cyanosis, jaundice, skin rashes and birth marks.

Head. Look for abnormalities in shape of the cranium, making allowance for the moulding that occurs during birth, and assess the tension of the anterior fontanelle and the width of the sutures. If the fontanelle feels unusually full or if there is more than 1 cm of sutural separation, hydrocephalus should be suspected and ultrasound examination performed.

Face. Look for signs of facial nerve palsy.

Eyes. Asymmetry of eye size is abnormal. It may mean that one eye is unusually small, due to congenital infection or developmental defect, or that the other eye is abnormally large, suggesting congenital glaucoma which is an emergency. The eye should be checked for signs of infection and the lenses for cataract. There is no need to perform retinoscopy routinely.

Nose. The nose is the baby's principal airway and should be checked for signs of obstruction.

Mouth. A baby will usually open its mouth if gentle downward pressure is applied to the chin. The palate should be inspected for clefts and palpated for submucosal clefts. The oral cavity should be checked for the presence of natal teeth, cysts or thrush (candida infection).

Jaw. An unusually small or recessed mandible can be a source of feeding difficulty or occasionally of respiratory obstruction.

Neck. The neck should be quickly palpated for signs of thyroid enlargement. A sternomastoid tumour is not usually present at birth.

Chest. There is little to be gained by routinely auscultating the lungs of babies who are pink and not breathless.

Heart. Note the side of the chest on which the apex is felt, and the forcefulness of the cardiac impulse. Heart murmurs at this age are very common and relate to the transition from fetal to adult circulatory pattern. It is difficult even for experienced cardiologists to sort out clinically significant murmurs from non-significant ones. It is important however not to generate widespread parental anxiety by investigating and following up all babies with a heart murmur. Selection can be improved by auscultating the heart at the second examination when many transitional murmurs will have disappeared. As a rule, soft, mid or early systolic murmurs are likely to be insignificant, whereas diastolic, pansystolic, or very loud murmurs are likely to be important.

Abdomen. The yield of positive findings from routine abdominal palpation is low. The liver edge is usually palpable about 2 cm below the right costal margin and the spleen can be tipped in at least 20% of normal babies. The lower poles of both kidneys may be palpable. It is worth checking that there is no bladder enlargement (which may indicate posterior urethral valves in male infants).

Groins. Ensure that both femoral pulses can be felt, as their absence may denote coarctation of the aorta. Check for hernias.

Genitalia. Check that the genitalia are clearly either male or female. In the male, check that the testes are in the scrotum and that the urethral meatus is where it should be. In the female, check that there is no bulging of the perineum or vulva, which may be due to imperforate hymen (Fig. 5.4) and remember that

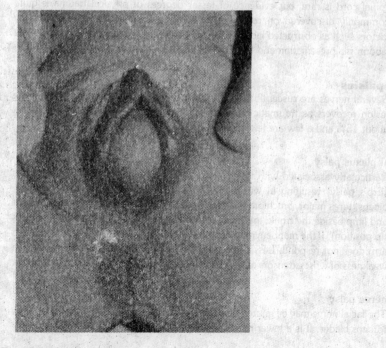

Fig. 5.4. Bulging imperforate hymen in hydrometrocolpos.

a little vaginal bleeding or discharge of clear mucus are both normal phenomena secondary to the influence of maternal and placental hormones.

Anus. Ask if the baby has passed meconium, and check that the anus is present and normally located. There is no need for routine rectal examination.

Spine. Turn the baby prone and look for scoliosis. The entire dorsal midline should be inspected for lumps, naevi, hairy patches, pits or sinuses each of which may be a surface indicator of spinal cord abnormality.

Hips. Examination of the hips (see p. 178) is best left to the end of the examination as it may upset the baby. The early diagnosis and management of congenital dislocation offers a much better prognosis than when diagnosis is delayed.

Central nervous system. A full neurological assessment of the newborn is time-consuming and demands considerable skill and experience. It is reasonable to limit the routine clinical examination to the detection of gross neurological abnormality, which can largely be excluded by observing the spontaneously moving baby while conducting the rest of the examination.

If it is considered that follow-up is needed the parents should receive a detailed explanation.

Biochemical screening. Routine screening on blood-spot tests is carried out for phenylketonuria and hypothyroidism. Some hospitals also screen for cystic fibrosis.

BIRTH INJURY (PHYSICAL TRAUMA)

In a modern obstetric unit serious birth injury, such as tearing of the dura or spinal cord is rare, but evidence of lesser degrees of physical trauma is quite commonly discovered on routine examination. Trauma is predisposed to by factors such as obstructed labour (due to small pelvis or large baby), precipitate labour, malpresentation and heroic instrumental delivery.

Nerve palsies

Several nerves are susceptible to traction or direct pressure injury. Usually the lesion recovers as traumatic swelling subsides, but minor disability persists in about 15% and a few are left handicapped.

Brachial plexus palsy

Particularly associated with large fetal size, it usually affects C5 and C6 roots (Erb's palsy) resulting in weakness or paralysis of deltoid, serratus anterior, biceps, teres major, brachioradialis and supinator. The affected arm lies straight and limp beside the trunk, internally rotated and with the fingers flexed (waiter's tip position). If the manoeuvre to elicit the Moro reflex is performed, the affected arm does not respond. Less commonly the lower roots are injured resulting in weakness of wrist extensors and intrinsic muscles of the hand (Klumpke's palsy).

Facial nerve palsy

The facial nerve may be injured by pressure from the maternal pelvic bones or by forceps blades. It is a lower motor neurone defect, usually unilateral.

Phrenic nerve palsy

Infrequently, the cervical roots of the phrenic nerve are damaged causing diaphragmatic paralysis and respiratory difficulty.

Sympathetic palsy

Damage to the first thoracic root may result in Horner's syndrome.

Skeletal injury

Skull fractures

The compliant skull of the newborn is remarkably resistant to fracture despite the considerable distortion that it undergoes. Asymptomatic linear fractures of the parietal bone are commonest, but depressed fractures sometimes occur and generally require surgical elevation.

Clavicle fracture

This is the most commonly seen fracture and occurs when there has been difficulty delivering the baby's shoulders. Complete breaks are painful and limit the baby's arm movements. Clavicle fractures heal well, but often with considerable callus formation.

Humerus and femur

Both fractures and epiphyseal injury may occur in these bones, usually during extremely difficult births.

Soft tissue injuries

Cephalhaematoma

In 1 or 2% of babies subperiosteal bleeding occurs, usually over the parietal bone, but occasionally occipitally when it may be mistaken for an encephalocele. The extent of the swelling, and therefore the amount of blood loss, is limited by the attachment of the periosteum to the margins of each skull bone. In 5% of cases, an associated linear skull fracture can be seen on X-ray. Cephalhaematomas require no treatment as the vast majority of them resolve spontaneously over a period of 1 to 2 months.

Subaponeurotic haemorrhage

In this case the haemorrhage occurs between the periosteum and galea aponeurotica, and, as the swelling is not limited in the same way as a cephalhaematoma, serious blood loss can occur. The routine prophylactic use of vitamin K has rendered this a very rare lesion.

Sternomastoid tumour

This is a fusiform fibrous mass which may be palpable, and visible, in the middle of the steromastoid muscle. It is commonly thought of as being secondary to trauma although the precise aetiology is uncertain. It is sometimes associated with cranial or facial asymmetry. The mass usually disappears over a period of about 6 months and gentle physiotherapy to prevent shortening of the muscle is usually the only treatment required.

Bruising and abrasions

Difficult births are often accompanied by bruising, which in breech delivery may be extensive. Usually there is little serious harm done to tissues although the breakdown of extravasated blood may contribute to neonatal jaundice. Skin abrasions are portals of entry for micro-organisms and should be carefully observed for signs of infection.

CONGENITAL MALFORMATIONS

Of all the causes of perinatal death, congenital abnormalities have shown the least decline over the years. Table 5.5 shows the main causes of perinatal mortality in relation to the current perinatal mortality rate of approx. 7.5 deaths per 1000 births.

Some authorities distinguish between *malformations*, which arise during embryogenesis and result from failure of normal development, and *deformations*, which arise later in gestation and result from mechanical constraint acting on normally formed organs and tissues. The latter include skull moulding, micrognathia (small jaw), postural foot deformities (p. 178) and congenital dislocation of the hip (p. 178). Oligohydramnios is commonly associated with deformations. Most of the common defects are described in the relevant chapter. Causation and prenatal diagnosis are discussed in Chapter 4.

At birth, most congenital defects can be detected by the routine newborn clinical examination (p. 58) or will present symptoms such as vomiting, cyanosis, jaundice or failure to pass urine or meconium. Some, however, especially in the cardiovascular system or renal tract, may escape detection. It is important to remember that multiple defects are quite common and the finding of one should always lead to a careful search for others (e.g. linked anorectal and renal anomalies, linked skeletal and cardiac anomalies). Constellations of defects may fit into recognized syndromes and every effort should be made to arrive at a diagnosis in these cases, as it may be possible to give a reasonably accurate prognosis and genetic risk of recurrence.

The problems of helping parents to cope with the bad news of a deformed baby are discussed in Chapter 2.

Table 5.5. Perinatal death rates by cause (per 1000 total births).

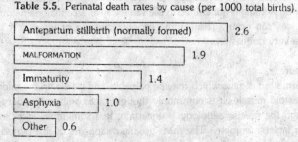

Antepartum stillbirth (normally formed)	2.6
MALFORMATION	1.9
Immaturity	1.4
Asphyxia	1.0
Other	0.6

BIRTHWEIGHT AND GESTATIONAL AGE CLASSIFICATION

Definitions (see also Fig. 5.5)

Low birthweight (lbw)—2500 g or less (in the UK applies to 7% of births)

Very low birthweight (vlbw)—1500 g or less (1% of UK births)

Extremely low birthweight—1000 g or less

Preterm—less than 37 completed weeks' gestation (two-thirds of lbw babies are preterm)

Term—37–41 weeks' gestation

Post-term—more than 41 weeks' gestation

Light for dates (lfd)—birthweight below 10th centile for sex and gestational age (one-third of lbw babies are lfd)

Heavy for dates (hfd)—birthweight above 90th centile for sex and gestational age

Appropriate for dates—birthweight between 10th and 90th centiles for sex and gestational age.

Although the relationship between birthweight and gestational age is generally good, almost all combinations of birthweight and gestational age can be found, from the extreme of the 4000 g 35-week gestation infant of the poorly controlled diabetic mother to the growth-retarded 2000 g, 42-week-gestation infant suffering from the effects of placental insufficiency (Fig. 5.6).

The correct classification of a baby in terms of gestational age is important, as maturity at birth is a major determinant of the ease with which a baby can adapt to extrauterine life. The correct classification in terms of weight for gestational age is also important, both as an indicator of underlying conditions, such as maternal diabetes, intrauterine infection or chromosome abnormality, and because light-for-dates babies are at risk for particular problems such as hypogly-

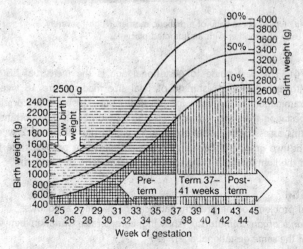

Fig. 5.5. Preterm babies (horizontal hatching) are of less than 37 weeks' gestation. Light-for-dates babies (vertical hatching) have a weight below the 10th centile for their gestation.

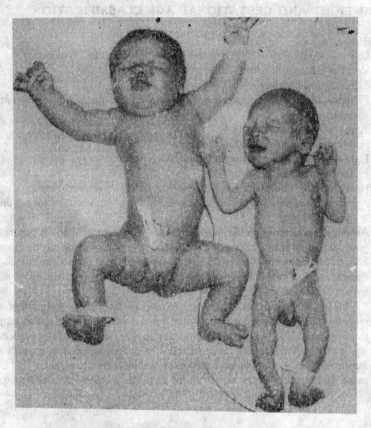

Fig. 5.6. (Left) typical obese baby of a diabetic mother. (Right) severely malnourished baby of a mother with an infarcted placenta.

caemia (p. 74). The best guide to gestational age is the menstrual history combined with an ultrasound estimate of fetal size made before 18 weeks' gestation. Examination of the baby for physical characteristics that correlate better with gestation than with size can also be helpful, but it is important to realize that this assessment is only accurate to within plus or minus 2 weeks (Fig. 5.7). The two groups of babies who present particular problems are the preterm, and the light-for-dates (who may be preterm, term or post-term).

The preterm baby

The principal problems of the preterm baby can be classified as follows:

System and organ immaturity (showing considerable variation between individuals of the same gestational age):

1 Respiratory distress syndrome.
2 Apnoeic spells.
3 Patent ductus arteriosus.

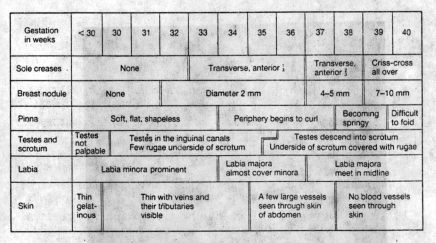

Gestation in weeks	< 30	30	31	32	33	34	35	36	37	38	39	40
Sole creases	None				Transverse, anterior ⅓				Transverse, anterior ⅔		Criss-cross all over	
Breast nodule	None			Diameter 2 mm					4–5 mm		7–10 mm	
Pinna	Soft, flat, shapeless				Periphery begins to curl				Becoming springy		Difficult to fold	
Testes and scrotum	Testes not palpable	Testes in the inguinal canals. Few rugae underside of scrotum				Testes descend into scrotum. Underside of scrotum covered with rugae						
Labia	Labia minora prominent				Labia majora almost cover minora				Labia majora meet in midline			
Skin	Thin gelatinous	Thin with veins and their tributaries visible				A few large vessels seen through skin of abdomen			No blood vessels seen through skin			

Fig. 5.7. The scoring of gestational age by physical features.

4 Intraventricular haemorrhage and other CNS damage.
5 Nutrition.
6 Infection.
7 Hyperbilirubinaemia.
8 Anaemia.
9 Hypothermia.
10 Renal function and fluid and electrolyte balance.

Lack of materno–fetal exchange during part or all of the third trimester of pregnancy:
1 Vitamin K deficiency.
2 Low immunoglobulin levels.
3 Low fat and carbohydrate stores.
4 Poorly mineralized skeleton.

Large surface area relative to body mass:
1 Hypothermia.
2 Fluid balance.

Respiratory distress syndrome (RDS)

This condition, also known as hyaline membrane disease because of its histological features, is virtually confined to preterm babies and is the most serious of the problems. It is mainly due to insufficient production of pulmonary surfactant, the normal function of which is to lower the surface tension at the interface between inspired gas and the liquid that lines the respiratory tract. Without surfactant the alveoli cannot be aerated efficiently. Additional defects in the premature respiratory system are structural immaturity of the lungs and chest wall, and poor respiratory drive. The end result is atelectasis, which disturbs gas exchange and gives rise to the X-ray appearance of diminished radiolucency and increased granularity (Fig. 5.8), and increased work of breathing, which, if it cannot be sustained, leads to carbon dioxide retention and often to apnoeic spells.

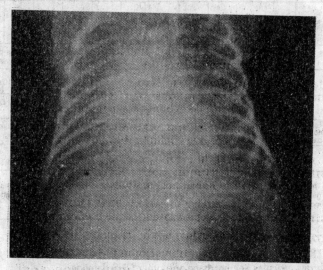

Fig. 5.8. Chest X-ray in RDS showing granularity and air bronchograms.

The signs of tachypnoea, inspiratory retraction of soft tissues in the intercostal spaces and epigastrium, and expiratory grunting are usually evident within minutes of birth and progress to cyanosis. A mixed acidosis due to lactate and carbon dioxide accumulation develops in more severe cases. Fortunately, lung function generally improves over a period of 3 to 7 days as surfactant production increases, and the management is to keep the baby alive and undamaged during this period. The mainstay of management is some form of assisted ventilation, combined with careful monitoring of physiological variables, especially arterial Po_2 (which may damage the developing retina if allowed to rise too high: a condition known as retinopathy of prematurity or retrolental fibroplasia). Death from respiratory failure should be very rare, although pulmonary complications and intraventricular haemorrhage are still major problems in very small infants.

Estimating the ratio of lecithin to sphingomyelin (the L:S ratio) in amniotic fluid enables some prediction of the risk of a baby developing RDS, and may help the obstetrician in planning elective preterm delivery.

There is now clear evidence that 48 hours of steroid therapy given to women in preterm labour reduces the likelihood and severity of RDS in their offspring and this therapy should be used whenever possible. There is also clear evidence for a beneficial effect of instilling either natural or synthetic surfactant into the trachea of preterm babies with RDS.

Patent ductus arteriosus (PDA)

The ductus arteriosus of the preterm infant often fails to close, especially when RDS is present. Left-to-right shunting causes pulmonary vascular congestion and pulmonary oedema which adds to the problem of gas exchange. The PDA can often be induced to close by giving a prostaglandin synthetase inhibitor such as indomethacin, but sometimes surgical closure is required.

Intraventricular haemorrhage and other forms of brain damage

In the walls of the lateral ventricles of preterm babies are fragile capillaries, from which bleeding may occur during birth asphyxia or in the course of RDS. Haemorrhage, which is demonstrated by cranial ultrasonography, may be local or extend into the ventricles or cerebral tissue. The more extensive the haemorrhage, the more likely are brain damage and hydrocephalus to occur. It is estimated that some degree of haemorrhage occurs in 40% of very small babies, although it causes serious damage in only a minority.

Another area of particular susceptibility in the brain of the preterm infant is the periventricular white matter which is prone to ischaemic injury, characteristically leading to spastic diplegia.

Nutrition

If the preterm newborn is to equal the fetal growth rate it requires approximately:

Energy	120 calories/kg/day
Water	120 ml/kg/day
Protein	3.5 g/kg/day
Fat	6 g/kg/day
Glucose	12 g/kg/day

If the baby is in good health, nutrients are given as milk, from breast or bottle if the baby can suck and swallow adequately, or else by gastric or jejunal tube. Daily volumes are increased to between 165 and 240 ml/kg according to the energy content of the milk and the baby's weight gain. Small frequent feeds, or even continuous infusions, are used. A growth rate of 12–15 g/kg/day is a reasonable target. For sick babies with RDS, intravenous nutrition is often safer until recovery occurs.

When enterally fed, preterm babies are susceptible to a bowel infection called necrotizing enterocolitis. The condition presents with abdominal distension, vomiting, and blood-stained stools. Oral feeds must be stopped, and appropriate antibiotic therapy started the moment the diagnosis is made if bowel resection is to be avoided.

Infection

Susceptibility to infection is even greater in the preterm than in the term infant (p. 75), and the general nature of the symptoms and signs makes diagnosis difficult.

Hyperbilirubinaemia

The common mechanisms for hyperbilirubinaemia in the preterm infant are an exaggeration of those responsible for physiological jaundice in the term infant (p. 73). However, preterm infants are more susceptible to bilirubin-induced brain damage.

Anaemia

Babies of all gestations reduce their erythropoietin production and allow their haemoglobin concentration to fall from the high levels appropriate to fetal life. In the preterm baby this fall is more pronounced, sometimes leading to symptomatic anaemia at around 6 to 8 weeks of age. This is the *early* anaemia of prematurity. It is not due to a deficiency of haematinics and cannot be prevented by iron supplementation. A *late* anaemia may occur at around 4 to 6 months of age as a result of the baby running out of iron. It can be prevented by iron supplementation from 6 to 10 weeks of age.

Temperature control

The preterm baby is likely to drop his body temperature if the environment is not carefully controlled. This susceptibility is due to:

1 Large surface area relative to body mass.
2 Little subcutaneous fat.
3 Extended posture exposing a large skin surface area.
4 Large insensible water, and therefore heat, loss.
5 Possibly, defective central temperature regulation.

Hypothermia increases oxygen consumption, predisposes to RDS and infection, and must be avoided by nursing small babies in incubators or under radiant heaters.

Fluid and electrolyte balance

Most aspects of renal function are relatively poor in the preterm baby, and this, coupled with a high but largely unmeasurable water loss through the very permeable skin, can lead rapidly to dehydration and electrolyte disturbance.

Management of the preterm infant

Preterm infants who are unwell are looked after in special care baby units (SCBU) or neonatal units as they are now often called (Fig. 5.9).

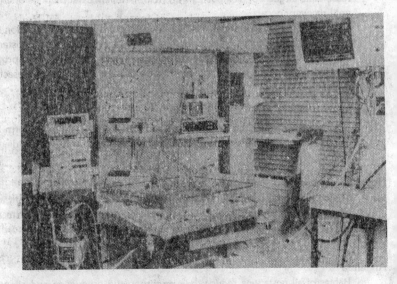

Fig. 5.9. A modern neonatal intensive care scene. The baby, beneath plastic sheeting to preserve humidity, looks diminutive among the hi-tech equipment.

Admission criteria to these units should be strict so that as few babies as possible are separated from their mothers. Parents must be allowed free access to their baby while on SCBU and every effort must be made to involve them in their baby's care as much as possible. Hospitals that do not have their own SCBU capable of providing long-term intensive care often transfer some cases to a Regional Unit where such facilities do exist. Babies travel quite well in expert hands. As a result of growing experience in the techniques of mechanical ventilation and supportive care, the mortality rate among preterm infants has fallen considerably and continues to do so. The survival rate for babies of less than 1500 g birthweight who are free of lethal malformation is currently better than 80%. This increased survival has yet to be fully evaluated in terms of quality but there seems to be no more than a 6–10% rate of serious handicap in this group.

The light-for-dates baby (Figs. 5.6 and 5.10)

By measuring length and head circumference in addition to weight it is possible to describe two extreme kinds of light-for-dates baby. Those whose length and head circumference are significantly higher on the centiles than their weight are said to be 'asymmetrically' growth retarded. This is classically the result of malnutrition late in gestation, usually due to pre-eclampsia. Those in whom all

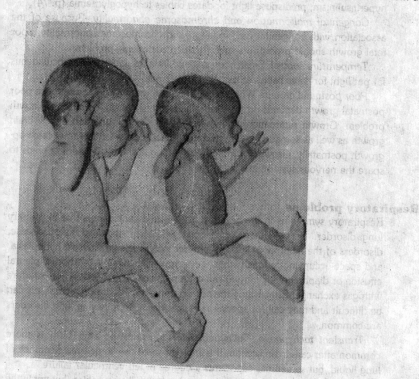

Fig. 5.10.   36-week gestation twins. The baby on the right shows quite severe symmetrical growth retardation.

three variables are more or less equally reduced are said to be 'symmetrically' growth retarded. These are either genetically small normal babies (in which case the term 'growth retarded' is inappropriate), genetically or chromosomally abnormal babies or else babies who have encountered adverse intrauterine environments, such as infection or drug effects, from an early stage of development. The special problems associated with light-for-dates are:

1 Perinatal asphyxia (especially asymmetric).
2 Hypoglycaemia (especially asymmetric).
3 Congenital malformation or chromosome abnormality (especially symmetric).
4 Poor postnatal growth (especially symmetric).
5 Hypothermia (both kinds).

Intrapartum asphyxia. Since avoidance of asphyxia depends heavily on a healthy placenta many light-for-dates babies are at particular risk. A paediatrician should be present at the birth of all fetuses expected to be light-for-dates. Intrapartum passage of meconium, especially common in term and post-term light-for-dates babies, carries the risk of meconium aspiration into the lung (see below).

Hypoglycaemia. Poor stores of carbohydrate and fat, and sometimes relative hyperinsulinism, predispose light-for-dates babies to hypoglycaemia (p. 74).

Congenital malformation and chromosome abnormality. Because of the association with congenital malformation and chromosome abnormality, poor fetal growth should prompt a search for such underlying problems.

Temperature control. Small body size and little insulation from subcutaneous fat put light-for-dates babies at risk of hypothermia.

Poor postnatal growth. Whether poor intrauterine growth continues as poor postnatal growth depends on the timing and severity of the intrauterine growth problem. Growth retardation evident before 20 weeks' gestation affects brain growth as well as somatic growth, and these babies often fail to show 'catch-up' growth postnatally. Growth retardation beginning in the third trimester tends to spare the nervous system, and subsequent growth is usually good.

Respiratory problems (other than RDS)

Respiratory symptoms in the newborn are by no means always due to primary lung disorder. Brain damage, metabolic acidosis, congenital heart disease, disorders of the diaphragm such as phrenic nerve palsy or muscle hypoplasia, and space-occupying lesions within the thorax such as pneumothorax, pleural effusion or diaphragmatic hernia, can each produce breathlessness and interfere with gas exchange. Establishing the correct cause for respiratory symptoms can be difficult and may call for special investigations. The following lung disorders are common:

Transient tachypnoea. Tachypnoea for a few hours after birth is more common after caesarean section. It is thought to be due to delayed clearance of lung liquid, but sometimes represents a degree of left ventricular failure.

Meconium aspiration. Intrapartum asphyxia in full-term babies (but not in the preterm) may cause intrapartum passage of meconium, which if inhaled can cause severe airway obstruction. The modern policy of clearing the upper airway and trachea of meconium at birth has reduced the incidence of this serious condition.

Congenital pneumonia. When micro-organisms invade the amniotic cavity before delivery the baby may be born with an established pneumonia. This is particularly likely to happen when there has been prolonged rupture of the membranes (longer than 24 hours). Group B streptococci and Gram-negative organisms such as *Escherichia coli* are most commonly incriminated.

Pneumothorax. One per cent of babies can be shown to have a pneumothorax on a chest X-ray taken shortly after birth. Occasionally this is symptomatic, and very occasionally drainage by thoracostomy tube is necessary.

Bronchopulmonary dysplasia (BPD). This is a chronic form of lung disease seen in some preterm babies who have been ventilated for severe RDS. It is due to lung damage by high oxygen concentration and high positive pressures. Steroid therapy is helpful in treatment but despite this some babies with BPD require prolonged oxygen therapy.

Metabolic problems

Hyperbilirubinaemia

In biochemical terms all babies develop hyperbilirubinaemia, and many are visibly jaundiced during the first week of life. The commonest mechanism is described as 'physiological' and reflects a temporary inadequacy in the system of conjugation during the switch from the fetal state, in which very little conjugation of bilirubin is desirable, to the neonatal state, when conjugation and hepatic excretion of bilirubin must take over from placental transfer. In term babies, the serum billirubin rarely exceeds 250 µmol/l and is usually normal by one week of age. In preterm babies, the rise in serum bilirubin continues for longer, peaks at a higher level, and takes a few more days to go. *Jaundice apparent within the first 24 hours is never physiological and strongly suggests excessive haemolysis.*

Unconjugated bilirubin (but not conjugated) can enter the nervous system and cause neuronal damage. The following factors make this more likely:

1 High serum bilirubin (greater than 400 µmol/l in the term baby, but lower levels in the preterm).
2 Preterm birth.
3 Acidosis.
4 Hypoxia.
5 Low serum albumin (to which bilirubin is normally bound).
6 Drugs that displace bilirubin from albumin (e.g. steroids).
7 Raised free-fatty acid levels (hypothermia, i.v. fat infusion).

The clinical syndrome of bilirubin encephalopathy (kernicterus) may result in death or serious handicap. When the rate of rise of serum bilirubin, and the presence of other risk factors, suggest that toxic levels may be reached, treatment with phototherapy is started. Phototherapy uses light of a wavelength that converts unconjugated bilirubin to non-toxic isomers which can be excreted without conjugation. Phototherapy takes time to work, however, and if a rapid fall in bilirubin is required an exchange transfusion must be performed.

The more common causes of pathological jaundice are as follows.

Increased bilirubin production (unconjugated jaundice):
1 Rhesus or ABO incompatibility.
2 Intrinsic red-cell defects leading to haemolysis.
3 Bruising.
4 Polycythaemia.

Defective hepatic conjugation (mainly unconjugated but may be mixed when there is an inflammatory process in the liver):
1 Hepatitis—due to congenital infection (p. 75).
2 Inborn errors of metabolism, e.g. galactosaemia (p. 220).
3 Hypothyroidism (p. 215).
4 Breast milk jaundice.
5 Hypoxia.
6 Sepsis.

Conjugated:
1 Biliary atresia.
2 Jaundice related to parenteral nutrition.

Haemolytic disease of the newborn

ABO incompatability is now the commonest cause of haemolytic jaundice, and usually occurs in a group A, but sometimes group B, baby of a group O mother. It occasionally requires an exchange transfusion. Rhesus haemolytic disease used to be the commonest cause of serious haemolysis, capable of causing profound jaundice and anaemia, and high output cardiac failure, but it is now rare due to the use of anti-D immunoglobulin. Breast milk jaundice is quite common, usually presenting as delayed resolution of physiological jaundice. Precise mechanisms are debated, but the milk of some mothers seems to interfere with conjugation. Hypothyroidism should always be considered when jaundice is slow to resolve, although the widespread introduction of screening for congenital hypothyroidism has reduced the risk of this important condition being missed.

Hypoglycaemia

At birth, the plentiful supplies of glucose that cross the placenta are cut off and the baby must maintain his own blood sugar from stored glycogen and fat until feeding is established. Glucose is an essential fuel for the nervous system, and hypoglycaemia, with symptoms of irritability, pallor, reluctance to feed and, more severely, seizures, rapidly leads to neuronal damage. The danger level for blood sugar is in the region of 1–1.5 mmol/l but every effort should be made to keep it at or above 2.5 mmol/l, by early and frequent milk feeds, which may be supplemented with glucose, or if necessary by i.v. infusion of dextrose.

The four groups at special risk of hypoglycaemia are the asymmetric light-for-dates, the preterm and the polycythaemic (due to the high utilization of glucose by red cells) baby and the infant of the diabetic mother (due to hyperinsulinism). In such cases, screening for hypoglycaemia with Dextrostix should be performed 4–6 hourly, until the risk of hypoglycaemia is passed.

Infant of a diabetic mother

The altered metabolic climate of the fetus of the established diabetic, gestational diabetic, or prediabetic mother can cause the following problems:

1 Large size and obesity relative to gestation.
2 Increased risk of RDS.
3 Hypoglycaemia, hypocalcaemia and jaundice.
4 Polycythaemia.
5 Congenital malformation, especially of lower body.

It has been shown that good diabetic control during pregnancy can greatly reduce these problems.

Hypocalcaemia

Hypocalcaemia (i.e. serum calcium below 1.7 mmol/l) may cause apnoea, neuromuscular excitability or seizures. It is most likely to arise in preterm infants, infants of diabetic mothers and following birth asphyxia. Hypocalcaemic seizures, unlike those of hypoglycaemia, have a good prognosis.

INFECTION

Fetal infection (Fig. 5.11)

Micro-organisms rarely succeed in crossing the placenta or penetrating the intact amnion. The effect of fetal infection depends on the nature of the organism, and the stage of gestation, with very early infections most likely to cause fetal death, abortion or major malformation.

Rubella. The rubella virus has a unique capability to cause malformation compatible with life, notably congenital heart defects, cataract and other ocular defects, sensorineural deafness and microcephaly with mental retardation. In addition, an infected baby may be born with evidence of active viraemia as shown by jaundice, hepatosplenomegaly, purpura and sometimes lesions of the bones and lungs. This 'extended rubella syndrome' can occur without malformation. A baby with congenital rubella may excrete live virus for several years. Congenital rubella is confirmed by isolation of virus from throat swabs or urine, by demonstrating rubella-specific IgM in the baby's blood or by persistence of rubella IgG antibody after the age of 8 months.

Cytomegalovirus (CMV). The incidence of congenital CMV infection is in the region of 3 or 4 cases per 1000 births. The brain and auditory pathway are the major targets for damage, which occurs in about 15% of infected fetuses. Only a small proportion of congenitally infected infants are symptomatic at birth. The diagnosis is made by isolation of the virus from throat swabs or urine or by detecting CMV specific antibody in the blood.

Toxoplasmosis. This disease is caused by a protozoon whose normal host is the cat. The incidence of fetal infection is though to be in the region of 3 per 1000 but may be higher. The signs are variable, but CNS involvement with hydroceph-alus and chorioretinitis are common. One-third of cases show signs of infection at

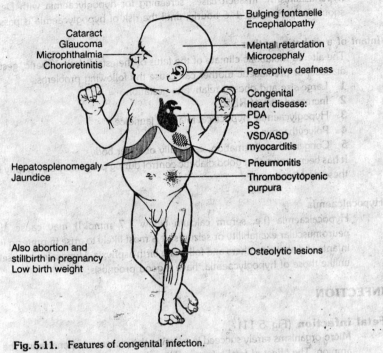

Fig. 5.11. Features of congenital infection.

birth, with hepatosplenomegaly, jaundice, purpura, chorioretinitis and abnormal CSF, but these signs may be delayed for weeks or months after birth.

Human immunodeficiency virus (HIV). Approximately 50–60% of infants of HIV seropositive mothers are prenatally or perinatally infected with HIV and this mode of transmission presently accounts for about 90% of AIDS infections in childhood. Symptoms and signs of AIDS may, rarely, be present at birth but more usually the diagnosis is made some time between 6 months and 2 years of age. As among infected adults, clinical manifestations are widespread and variable although an all too common mode of presentation in children is progressive encephalopathy. The number of AIDS cases in babies and young children is increasing year by year at an alarming rate.

Hepatitis B infection. Between 70–90% of mothers who are hepatitis B antigen positive, and whose serum contains 'e' antigen but not 'e' antibody, will transmit the virus to their offspring unless steps are taken to prevent it. Excellent protection can be achieved by giving babies at risk a combination of passive immunity with hepatitis B immune globulin and active immunity with hepatitis B vaccine. Babies of mothers whose serum contains 'e' antibody should receive just hepatitis B vaccine.

Syphilis, tuberculosis and malaria can cause fetal infection; all three are rare in the UK.

Intrapartum infection

When the membranes rupture the fetus may be invaded by the flora of the birth canal. The following infections are particularly likely to be acquired in this way:

1 Gonoccocal ophthalmia.
2 *Candida albicans* infection.
3 *Herpes simplex.*
4 Pneumonia and/or meningitis due to group B streptococci or *Listeria monocytogenes.*

Infection acquired after birth

Once born, the baby rapidly becomes colonized by bacteria and usually this occurs without harm. Infection is especially likely if colonization is heavy or if the organisms are of high pathogenicity. A poor local inflammatory response predisposes to bacteraemia and septicaemia, and from the blood stream organisms may lodge in deep tissue to give rise to meningitis, osteomyelitis or pneumonia. The common early signs of sepsis in the newborn are:

1 Lethargy and hypotonia.
2 Poor feeding, abdominal distension or vomiting.
3 Pallor and mottling of the skin.
4 Disturbed temperature regulation.
5 Apnoeic spells.

Any baby suspected of being infected should be carefully examined and promptly investigated with blood culture, chest X-ray, microscopy and culture of urine and CSF, and surface swabs. Broad-spectrum antibiotic therapy is started pending the results of the tests. Among the commonest organisms causing serious infection are the Gram-negative organisms (such as *E. coli*, Serratia, and Pseudomonas), *Staphylococcus pyogenes*, coagulase-negative staphylococci and group B haemolytic streptococci.

Sticky eye

The cause of most sticky eyes is poor drainage down the nasolacrimal duct. Often no organisms are isolated and all that is necessary is to gently bathe the conjunctivae with warm saline. More serious eye infections may be due to staphylococci, occasionally *Chlamydia trachomatis* or the gonococcus. In these cases, prompt isolation of the organism and specific therapy are essential.

Skin infection

Septic spots and paronychia, usually due to staphylococcal infection, are relatively common and responsive to local treatment—though there should be no hesitation in using systemic antibiotics if the infection is severe or the baby seems unwell.

Candidal infection

Infection of the oral cavity and nappy area by yeasts is common but responds well to nystatin or miconazole. Therapy should be continued for one week longer than it takes to clear the signs of infection, and if a dummy has been used it should be discarded.

Convulsions

Convulsions occurring in the first 48 hours of life are usually due to intrapartum brain damage and are generally a bad prognostic sign. Other causes of seizures are meningitis, hypoglycaemia, hypocalcaemia, hypomagnesaemia, hypo- or hypernatraemia, and inborn errors of metabolism.

Seizures always require immediate and thorough investigation and therapy of any underlying disorder. If the cause cannot be remedied, anticonvulsant medication is given.

FURTHER READING

Chiswick M. *Neonatal Medicine*. Update Publications.
Fleming P, Speidel B and Dunn P. *A Neonatal Vade-mecum*. Lloyd Luke Medical Books.
Harper PS. *Practical Genetic Counselling*. Wright.
Milner RDG and Herber SM. *A Colour Atlas of the Newborn*. Wolfe Medical Publications.
Roberton C. *Textbook of Neonatology*. Churchill Livingstone.
Schaffer AJ and Avery MA. *Diseases of the Newborn*. WB Saunders.
Vulliamy DC. *The Newborn Child*. Churchill Livingstone.

Chapter 6
Nutrition

Mens sana in corpore sano. Good nutrition is the foundation stone of healthy growth which in turn facilitates healthy development. Worldwide, the only common nutritional problem is starvation. In industrialized societies the main problems are eating unwisely or too much.

Nutrition is particularly important in the first year of life when the infant is entirely dependent on his carers to feed him. Babies treble their birth weight in the first year of life; to treble it again takes 10 years. Furthermore, 65% of total postnatal brain growth take place in the first year of life. Starvation may permanently hamper both physical and mental development. Average nutritional requirements during the first year of infancy are:

water	150 ml/kg/day;
calories	110 kcal/kg/day;
vitamin C	15 mg/day;
vitamin D	400 i.u./day (10 µg cholecalciferol);
calcium	600 mg/day ⎫ average during first year
iron	6 mg/day ⎭

Milk

Milk is a poor source of iron but is rich in calcium and calories (400 per 560 ml or 1 pint). There is little fat-soluble vitamin D in human milk, but substantial amounts of water-soluble vitamin D sulphate. The main differences in composition between human and cow's milk are shown in Table 6.1.

It will be noted that in cow's milk the protein content is much higher and most of it is casein: the lactose content is lower: the fat content is similar, but more of it is in the form of saturated fatty acids. The sodium (and potassium) content is higher, leading to a higher osmolality. The phosphorus content is higher. The processing of cow's milk alters the protein so that reconstituted dried or evaporated milks are more easily digested by infants than is fresh cow's milk.

Table 6.1. Differences between human and cow's milk.

	Human milk (per 100 ml)	Cow's milk (per 100 ml)
Protein:	1.2 g	3.3 g
casein	0.3 g	2.7 g
soluble proteins	0.9 g	0.6 g
Lactose	7.0 g	4.8 g
Fat:	3.7 g	3.7 g
saturated	48%	58%
unsaturated	52%	42%
Sodium	15 mg	58 mg
Phosphorus	15 mg	100 mg

Doorstep milk should not be given to infants under 6 months. From 6 to 12 months of age it may be given, but it must be boiled first if it is not pasteurised, home conditions are poor or there is no refrigerator.

Strenuous attempts have been made to formulate infant feeds to approximate closely to breast milk in regard to protein, lactose, fat, sodium and phosphorus content. These modern milks are fortified with vitamins and iron (the bioavailability of this iron is not as good as that in breast milk).

A *full-strength* feed is made up according to the instructions on the container: a *half-strength* feed is made up with double the usual amount of water.

Breast feeding

Successful breast feeding requires the active participation of both parties. The baby needs well-established sucking and swallowing reflexes and a good appetite. These are normally present in the healthy, full-term infant but may be defective in the sick or preterm infant. The mother needs a good draught reflex, which may take a little while to develop with a first baby. The stimulus to this reflex initially is contact of the baby with the nipple, but later the baby's hunger cry, or even thinking about the baby, may be sufficient. The response is a secretion by the posterior pituitary of oxytocin which causes contraction of the myoepithelial cells around the alveoli of the breast, with ejection of milk down the ducts to the ampulla. In the puerperium, the oxytocin secreted will also cause uterine contraction, and midwives traditionally used to put the newborn baby straight to the breast to encourage expulsion of the placenta. For the same reason, breast feeding may be associated with abdominal cramps in the first week or two.

Breast-fed babies may be fed by the clock (usually every 4 hours) or on demand. Regular weighing is the only means of knowing whether the milk supply is adequate. Crying does not necessarily mean hunger; sleep does not necessarily mean satiation. Breast feeding can be a highly satisfying experience for the mother and ensures close physical contact between mother and infant. There is, however, no evidence to suggest that bottle-fed babies are either nutritionally or emotionally deprived.

Infant feeding practices seem to be dictated largely by fashion. Mothers may feel that breast feeding limits their social activities, spoils their clothes or ruins their figures. Rich families in past ages employed wet nurses (e.g. Exodus, 2 vii): today the bottle is more readily available. There are many good reasons for encouraging mothers to breast feed, and the encouragement should start no later than the antenatal clinic. Breast milk is nutritionally ideal for at least 4 months in the full-term baby. It is inexpensive, readily available, and convenient. Breast-fed babies are less prone to gastroenteritis, infantile eczema, obesity, hypocalcaemic fits and hypernatraemic states.

Protection from infection results not only from the reduced opportunity to contaminate the milk. Maternal antibody in breast milk discourages colonization of the gut by pathogens. The pH of breast milk and the presence of certain substances, including lactoferrin and bifidus factor, encourage colonization of the bowel with lactobacilli rather than coliforms. Breast feeding, even for a month, gives an infant an excellent start to life. Nobody wants to see unwilling mothers browbeaten into breast feeding, but there is a happy mean between that and the total indifference shown by many doctors and nurses. Experience has shown repeatedly that mothers will respond to information, advice and encouragement.

Many drugs are excreted in breast milk but maternal medication is only exceptionally a contra-indication to breast feeding. Nor is 'breast milk jaundice' a reason to stop.

Bottle feeding

Bottle feeding offers opportunities to infect the baby, and the preparation of feeds and sterilization of bottles must therefore be meticulous. Bottles and teats may be sterilized by boiling or by immersion in hypochlorite solution: by either method, attention to detail is crucial. Evaporated milks are sterile, and dried milks pathogen-free, until the tins are opened. Feeds should normally be made up according to the manufacturer's directions and should be given either 4-hourly or on demand. The newborn baby will require feeding round the clock, but within a few weeks will drop the night feed. So long as a night feed is demanded, it must be given. Leaving him to cry is pointless and unkind.

Attention to detail in making up the feed is as essential as detail in sterilizing bottles. The scoop appropriate to the milk powder should be used, it should be filled without compressing the powder (unless otherwise stated) and should be levelled off with a knife. Additional scoops, heaped scoops, packed scoops or additional cereal should be avoided. They add extra calories which encourage obesity, and extra solutes which cause thirst and irritability. It is conventional to warm infant feeds to approximately body temperature, but many babies will accept feeds direct from the refrigerator and come to no harm.

Mixed feeding

The term 'weaning' is variously used to mean taking the baby off the breast or introducing solid foods and is therefore best avoided. The age at which foods other than milk are introduced has been influenced to some extent by fashion. A full-term baby will not develop any nutritional deficiency within 4 months of birth. Mixed feeding should start at 4–6 months.

The main principles of mixed feeding are as follows:

1 Ensure an adequate introduction of food containing protein and iron: avoid excess carbohydrate (e.g. cereals and sugar).
2 Introduce one new food at a time, starting with very small quantities and increasing gradually if the food is accepted and tolerated.
3 If a new food is not accepted by the infant, try something else. Later feeding difficulties may stem from misguided insistence on an infant taking food that he does not enjoy.

As the semi-solid component of the diet is increased, the number and volume of milk feeds should be decreased. The duration of breast feeding rarely exceeds 6 months in Western societies, but averages 2 years or more in developing countries. The average 1-year-old will be having three main meals a day, with a small drink or snack mid-morning, mid-afternoon and at bedtime.

Vitamin supplements

Infants need 400 i.u. vitamin D and 15 mg vitamin C daily. These may be provided by fortified baby milks, but must otherwise be supplied as vitamin drops given for the first year or two of life. Small preterm babies may need slightly bigger doses initially. Asian children may need to take a vitamin D supplement for longer.

For older children a good, balanced diet will meet their needs for vitamins. The principal food sources of the most important vitamins are:

1 Vitamin C: citrus and other fruits, potatoes, vegetables.
2 Vitamin D: margarine, non-white fish, liver (including fish livers).
3 Riboflavin: liver and kidney, yeast extract (e.g. Marmite).
4 Folic acid: liver and kidney, leaf vegetables.

Nutrition of toddlers and schoolchildren

Changing social patterns in industrialized countries have had profound influences, not necessarily beneficial, on the nutrition of children. A tradition of home cooking, home baking and indeed home growing of some fresh vegetables has given place to supermarket shopping, fast foods, convenience foods, takeaway meals and eating out. Even in times and places of high unemployment this tends to persist. If father loses his job, mother may seek work outside the home, and although more men are competent cooks today than even a decade ago, many families continue to buy food that needs little more than heating up.

Recent concerns about food additives—artificial flavourings, colourings, sweeteners, preservatives—and food allergies have turned many families towards 'natural' food and a return to home cooking.

The chief nutritional requirements of children are protein for building new tissue as they grow, and sufficient fat and carbohydrate to meet their substantial energy needs. The requirements for first-class protein (egg, milk, fish, meat) are about 1–1.5 g/kg/day. Energy requirements average 110 kcal/kg/day and are made up of three components:

	kcal/kg/day
Maintenance	80
Growth	5
Physical activity	25
Total	110

The relationships between diet and the degenerative disorders of adult life will doubtless be debated for decades to come. The dietary basis of obesity, dental caries and much constipation in childhood is less complex. Refined sugar should be eaten in moderation, and sticky sweets preferably not at all. An excess of fried foods (e.g. fish and chips) encourages obesity. Fibre helps prevent constipation. Most fizzy drinks ('pop'), so loved by children, have little or no nutritional value and help to rot teeth. Milk is highly nutritious but at 400 kcal/pint an excessive intake can be a major contribution to obesity.

FEEDING PROBLEMS

Difficulties with feeding are common. In very young infants they may be to do with bottles, but at all ages they are more often to do with battles. Feeding mismanagement in early life may present with vomiting, disturbed bowel habit, unsatisfactory weight gain or crying. Most difficulties arise from one or more of three faults:

1   The *quantity* of food is wrong. Both underfeeding and overfeeding may lead to vomiting and crying. In the first, weight gain is consistently poor. An overfed baby gains weight excessively to begin with, but may later lose. Overfeeding is particularly common in bottle-fed babies, partly because they are often fed to the limit of their capacity, partly because food has a sedative effect, and partly because of the mistaken belief that the biggest babies are the best.

2   The *kind* of food is wrong. Excessively early mixed feeding may lead to vomiting, diarrhoea and crying. A return to a milk diet will allow recovery, followed by cautious reintroduction of solids. Changing from one milk to another rarely achieves anything.

3   The feeding *technique* is wrong. This is a common cause of difficulties and can only be recognized by watching the baby feeding. The baby may not be held comfortably: the bottle may be held at the wrong angle; the hole in the teat may be too small or too big: the milk may have been wrongly prepared. Instruction and advice provide the remedy.

One particular form of crying in early infancy deserves special mention. *Three-months colic*, or evening colic, is a very common problem arising in early life and lasting, as a rule, not beyond the age of 3 months. An otherwise placid baby devotes one part of the day, most commonly between the 6 pm. and 10 pm feeds, to incessant crying. He may or may not stop when picked up, but certainly cries again if put down. Attention to feeds, warmth, wet nappies, etc., are unavailing. Theories abound but the cause is unknown.

It has been suggested that at any feed an infant needs to achieve a certain amount of food and a certain amount of sucking. Babies vary in their need for sucking time. Most babies take a feed in 20–30 minutes, but some drain their bottle in 5–10 minutes and may then have filled their stomachs without satisfying their need to suck. Such an infant may solve his own problems by discovering how to suck his thumb. The widespread use of comforters (dummies) in the face of sometimes vehement opposition from the medical and nursing professions suggests that mothers have known this for a long time. Since comforters will continue to be used, just as fireworks will continue to be made and sold, it may be more constructive to stop trying to abolish them and instead try to ensure that they are used safely. Their only hazard is as a vehicle for infection: they do not make teeth protrude.

Feeding difficulties after 6 months may result from allowing unsuitable foods, but with increasing age they more commonly result from attempts to insist on the child eating foods that he dislikes. There is a delicate distinction between encouraging the conservative child to try something new, and coercing the reluctant child to eat 'what is good for him'. The mother who sits by the high chair supplying endless diversions whilst she subtly spoons in 'one for Sarah, one for Teddy', is more likely to be storing up trouble than solving a problem. The management of such problems lies in the patient, repeated but firm explanation that no normal child with access to food will starve: that children of some ages are dominated by the need for food, but at other ages it may be a low priority; that wise parents do not start battles with their children that they are bound to lose; and that a mother will often achieve most by doing least.

Some groups of children present inherent problems with feeding. Preterm babies make no demands and must be fed by the clock. Some mentally retarded children are also abnormally placid and cannot be demand fed: they may also have sucking and swallowing difficulties. Physically handicapped children, especially those with cerebral palsy, may be very difficult to feed because of muscular weakness and incoordination.

Obesity

Obesity in childhood is a common and troublesome problem—troublesome to the child, the family and the doctor. Some heavy-weight newborns seem to have insatiable appetites: their price for peace is food, and they seem doomed to obesity from the womb (Fig. 6.1). In others, the tendency to excessive weight gain may appear in infancy, toddlerhood or during school years. Although only 10–20% of obese infants are still fat when they start school, half of all fat schoolchildren were overweight as babies. Fat children often come from fat families. Many fat children are undoubtedly gluttons, tucking away excessive

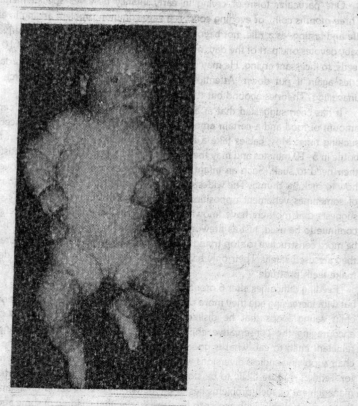

Fig. 6.1. An obese 3-month-old baby weighing 8.2 kg.

calories, predominantly from carbohydrates. Equally certainly, some fat children do not eat excessively but have an abnormal tendency to lay down fat. Similarly, some fat children take a lot of exercise, others none. Obese children are nearly always tall for their age. Obesity combined with short stature suggests a possible endocrine cause.

Obesity may limit exercise tolerance; associated knock-knee may lead to complaints of leg pains; and in boys the disappearance of the penis into a pad of suprapubic fat may lead to a mistaken diagnosis of hypogonadism. The dominant symptoms, however, are psychological. The fat child may be teased and ostracized, and the fat girl cannot buy fashionable clothes. There is good evidence that fat children tend to become fat adults, and weight reduction is advisable. The patients and their families are often ambivalent about dieting: they would like to lose weight, but not with sufficient zeal to endure the inconvenience.

For most children, a 1000 calorie diet, encouragement to exercise, and ample moral support form the basis of treatment. Group activities may help. Drugs are best avoided; amphetamines should not be prescribed. Any emotional stresses at home or at school should if possible be alleviated. If satisfactory weight loss is achieved, follow-up should not be too short. If necessary, admission to hospital allows the strict supervision of a more restricted diet and weight is rapidly lost. Sadly, it is often regained rapidly after returning home. Finally, obesity is almost never due to endocrine disease and parents need to be told that the child's 'glands are alright'.

DEFECTIVE NUTRITION

Nutritional deficiency may consist in a general shortage of food or in lack of specific dietary factors. Overall food deficency is only seen in Britain in children who have been grossly neglected, but in many parts of the world, especially the tropics and subtropics, *infantile marasmus* is all too common. In these areas, breast-feeding is customarily continued for about 2 years, and there is very little alternative. If the supply of breast milk is inadequate, starvation ensues. The infant with marasmus is a prey to intercurrent infection, and mortality is high. There is also evidence that starvation in the first year of life, even if subsequently corrected, may cause permanent mental handicap.

Kwashiorkor, or protein energy malnutrition, is seen in the same parts of the world as marasmus but in older children, usually 2–4 years old. At this age the next baby often displaces the older sibling from the breast, and in many places it is customary to send the older child away to stay with relatives after the new baby has arrived. Food deprivation may therefore coincide with emotional disturbance, and the characteristic picture of kwashiorkor develops. The child is listless, the face, limbs and abdomen swell, the hair is sparse and dry, and there are areas of hyperpigmentation ('black enamel paint') especially on the legs. Diarrhoea is sometimes a feature.

An increasing number of Western families are adopting bizarre diets in the name of religion or conservation. Growing children fed on such diets may be malnourished. That contrasts with standard vegetarianism; children in vegetarian families are healthy (and most unlikely to be obese).

Worldwide, vitamin deficiencies remain an appalling problem for the world's children. It is estimated that at least 250 000 young children go blind each year from xerophthalmia and that nearly 10 million suffer from lesser degrees of that same vitamin A deficiency. In western countries vitamin deficiencies have become relatively rare.

Rickets

Nutritional rickets results from dietary deficiency of vitamin D coupled with inadequate exposure to sunlight. It is quite common in Asian children in the UK because their traditional diet is poor in calcium and they receive little sunlight on their skins. It presents at times of active growth—in the first 3 years of life and at puberty.

Rickets may complicate malabsorption states and certain rare forms of renal disease. Normal bone formation requires a proper balance of calcium and phosphorus in the tissues, especially at the epiphyses where active growth is most rapid. Vitamin D is involved in the absorption of calcium from the gut and in the deposition of normal bone. Deficiency of calcium, phosphorus or vitamin D interferes with bone maturation beyond the stage of provisional calcification which therefore tends to accumulate as osteoid tissue. This accounts for the thickening of epiphyses seen particularly at the wrists, ankles and costochondral junctions ('rickety rosary'). The frontal bones may also be thickened. Toddlers develop bow legs: older children become knock-kneed. There is hypotonia.

In nutritional rickets the serum calcium is normal or reduced and the alkaline phosphatase is raised. X-rays show broadening, cupping and rarefaction of the bone ends (Fig. 6.2). In malabsorption states rickets is liable to develop after treatment has been started because it is a disease of growing bones. Vitamin D supplements should therefore be given.

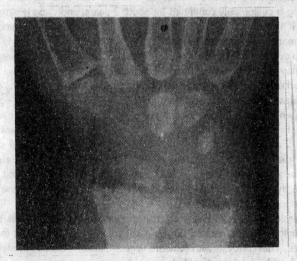

Fig. 6.2.   X-ray of wrist showing rickets.

Rickets may complicate renal disease under two quite different circumstances both of which are rare. *Glomerular* renal rickets may complicate chronic renal failure mainly because of the failure of the normal conversion in the kidney of 25-hydroxycholecalciferol to the active 1,25-dihydroxycholecalciferol. *Tubular* renal rickets results from a failure of normal tubular reabsorption of phosphate and may be a feature of many inborn errors of tubular function including vitamin D-resistant rickets and cystinosis. The rickets sometimes seen in children taking long-term anticonvulsants (especially phenytoin or barbiturates) is thought to be of renal origin.

The prevention of nutritional rickets can be assured by a daily vitamin D intake of 400 i.u. throughout infancy and early childhood. All baby milk foods and most cereals have vitamin D added. Infants are therefore likely to obtain sufficient from their diet, but preterm babies should be given drops of vitamin concentrate for 6 months. The treatment of established cases requires the education of the mother regarding the diet, and supplementary vitamin D, 5000 i.u. daily, until X-rays show healing. Excessive doses are dangerous. Renal rickets is more difficult to treat and requires careful and continuous metabolic control.

Scurvy

Scurvy is now a very rare disease amongst children in the UK. It is also rare in countries where malnutrition is prevalent because fruit is usually plentiful. In infancy the recommended vitamin C intake is 15 mg daily, although scurvy will probably not develop on half this amount. The predominant symptom of scurvy is haemorrhage, which may occur into the gums, the skin or subperiosteally. X-rays show periosteal elevation and, later, calcification of subperiosteal haemorrhages. There is a rapid response to vitamin C.

FURTHER READING

Francis D. *Nutrition for Children.* Blackwell Scientific Publications.
McLaren D and Burman D. *Textbook of Paediatric Nutrition.* Churchill Livingstone.
Wood CBS and Walker Smith JA. *MacKeith's Infant Feeding and Feeding Difficulties.* Churchill Livingstone.

Chapter 7
Abnormal Growth and Sex Development

ABNORMAL GROWTH

Failure to thrive

The term is applied to a child in the first year or two of life whose predominant symptom is unsatisfactory weight gain. The main causes are as follows:

1. Inadequate food intake:
   (a) feeding mismanagement or neglect;
   (b) poor appetite;
   (c) mechanical problems, e.g. cleft palate, cerebral palsy.
2. Vomiting:
   (a) pyloric stenosis, hiatus hernia;
   (b) feeding mismanagement;
   (c) food intolerance.
3. Defects of digestion or absorption:
   (a) cystic fibrosis;
   (b) food intolerance (including coeliac disease);
   (c) chronic infective diarrhoea.
4. Failure of utilization:
   (a) chronic infections;
   (b) heart failure, renal failure;
   (c) metabolic disorders.
5. Emotional deprivation.

It is sometimes possible to recognize quickly the main reason for failing to thrive—there may be a clear history of inadequate food intake or of chronic food loss by way of vomiting or diarrhoea. Sometimes physical examination including a check on the urine reveals an obvious cause. However, it is common for no clear reason to be apparent at the first consultation: the child appears to have caring and competent parents who offer enough food and they do not provide a dramatic story suggesting any particular disorder. Solving the problem is a difficult art, for the range of possibilities is large and no one wants to embark on massive overinvestigation. If possible a weight record card, perhaps from the Child Health Centre at the time of immunizations, will reveal previous weights from which one can deduce when the failure to thrive began. The health visitor should be able to provide a reliable account of the state of the home and whether both food and emotional nourishment are available there. A home visit can be most revealing. Sometimes the initial enquiries and checks are negative and it is necessary to admit the child to hospital to be fed standard amounts of food and observed to see if weight gain occurs, and whether there is any diarrhoea or vomiting. At the same time basic screening tests can be performed on the blood and urine to exclude infection and other common disorders. If these tests are negative, and the child is still failing to thrive, tests for rarer disorders including the syndromes of malabsorption become mandatory.

Short stature

The majority of children for whom medical advice is sought because of short stature are normal, short children. Some of them were born light-for-dates and many have short relatives including one or both parents. Their *rate of growth* is normal, as shown by serial measurements plotted on a centile chart. More accurately the growth velocity can be measured over 6–12 months by dividing a height increment by the time elapsed; these measurements can be plotted on a growth velocity chart. A child's growth velocity should be about the mean on that chart; if not the child is growing abnormally compared with his peers. The commonest reason for a child being short is having short parents, because the child's height centile will be approximately the mean of his parents' centiles for height. Delayed puberty (often familial) and delayed bone age are common with short stature; the later pubertal growth spurt allows these children to catch up. If serial observations of height show an abnormally slow rate of increase, some other explanation must be sought. The main causes of pathological short stature are:

1 Defects of nutrition, digestion or absorption.
2 Social and emotional deprivation.
3 Most malformation syndromes.
4 Chronic disease (e.g. renal insufficiency).
5 In girls, abnormalities of the X chromosome (e.g. XO).
6 Deficiency of thyroid or growth hormone.
7 Long-term high-dose steroid therapy.
8 Disorders of bone growth (e.g. skeletal dysplasias).

Congenital hypothyroidism is likely to be recognized by neonatal screening or from other symptoms and signs (p. 215), but acquired hypothyroidism in older children commonly presents with short stature. Growth hormone deficiency may be isolated or part of a wider pituitary insufficiency, and it may be complete or partial. Growth hormone response to standardized exercise is a useful screening test, but for definitive diagnosis more complex tests (e.g. response to hypoglycaemia) are necessary. Bone age is retarded in both pituitary and thyroid deficiency, but especially in hypothyroidism.

Catch-up growth is a phenomenon that is seen in young children in whom the cause of retarded growth has been removed or corrected. There is immediate growth acceleration followed by gradual deceleration to a normal growth velocity as the appropriate growth centile is reached (Fig. 7.1). For infants and young children catch-up growth can be complete: thus a 4-year-old whose growth has been suppressed by massive doses of prednisolone will regain normal height once the steroid therapy is decreased or stopped. However, as puberty nears catch-up growth tends to be incomplete so that some degree of permanent stunting may occur from temporary factors which have stunted growth at that time.

Tall stature

Children who are entering puberty early or who are overweight tend to be relatively tall (90–97th centile). Children with heights well above the 97th centile

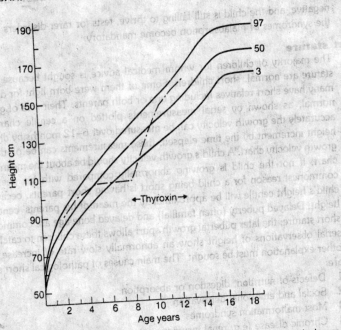

Fig. 7.1. Catch-up growth. This boy developed hypothyroidism which was diagnosed at the age of 8. With replacement therapy he had regained his appropriate height centile by the age of 11.

usually come from tall families. Formulae exist by which to calculate an approx imate final height from present height, age and bone age (or, more crudely, from parental heights). If it seems likely that height is going to exceed sociall acceptable limits and be an embarrassment, hormone therapy is exceptionall used to finish the growth process prematurely. This requires careful consideratio of career and recreational aspirations (ballet or basketball?).

Rarer causes of very tall stature include Klinefelter's syndrome (p. 91) an Marfan's syndrome. True Marfan's syndrome is an autosomal dominant disord of connective tissue characterized by long, slender habitus, arachnodactyl typical facial appearance and a propensity to dislocated lenses, prolapsing mit valve and dissecting aneurysm of the aorta. There are also 'marfanoid' famili and individuals who are long and thin but not liable to complications.

ABNORMAL SEX DEVELOPMENT

Intersex

The term is used to describe conditions in which the external genitalia at birth not clearly appropriate to one sex or the other but show features of both. So affected infants are masculinized genetic females; others are incompletely m culinized genetic males. The diagnostic problem is extremely urgent, pa because the most common underlying disorder is a dangerous one—the adre genital syndrome (p. 217)—and partly because prolonged uncertainty about the true sex is intolerable for the parents. Equally, much harm may be done if the wrong sex is assigned; later reversal may be traumatic. The 'right' sex is determined more by anatomy (functional possibilities) than by genetics.

Apart from the adrenogenital syndrome, causes of intersex are rare. True hermaphrodites (with ovarian and testicular tissue) may have indeterminate genitalia. Investigation of intersex begins with karyotyping and appropriate steroid chemistry.

Testicular feminization syndrome

In this rare but interesting condition there is a metabolic block in the activation of androgens in the tissues. Affected individuals are genetic males with testicles, but the external genitalia are of a female pattern. Sometimes testes are palpable in the labia majora, or may be found at the time of operation for inguinal hernia. In some patients normal female secondary sexual characteristics develop at puberty if the testes are left *in situ*, but orchidectomy is advised later because of a definite risk of malignant change. The condition is due to a recessive gene and there is therefore a recurrence risk of 25% amongst siblings.

Sex chromosome anomalies

These usually result from non-disjunction of sex chromosomes during gameto-genesis in one or other parent. They disturb the development of the gonad much more than they influence the development of the external genitalia and therefore rarely present before puberty except in the case of Turner's syndrome. Most children with abnormal sex chromosomes have normal external genitalia; most children with abnormal genitals (p. 90) have normal sex chromosomes.

Turner's syndromes (gonadal dysgenesis)

The characteristic karyotype is 45XO (one X chromosome is lacking) but deletions or mosaicism involving the X chromosome may also be found. It occurs in 1 out of every 2500 female babies. At birth the only noticeable abnormality may be lymphoedema of the legs, but later on the main features become more obvious and include short stature, webbed neck (pterygium colli), broad chest with wide-spaced nipples, and an increased carrying angle at the elbows (cubitus valgus) (Fig. 7.2). Pigmented naevi are common. In some cases there are coarctation of the aorta and urinary tract malformations. Secondary sexual characteristics usually do not appear; the uterus and vagina may be small and the gonads are represented by rudimentary streaks in the edge of the broad ligament. Breast development and menstrual periods may be induced by hormone therapy. Affected individuals remain infertile and short (few exceed 1.5 m or 5 feet) but growth hormone may improve stature at least in the short term.

Klinefelter's syndrome

The characteristic karyotype is 47XXY, but mosaicism may be found. Although this condition occurs in 1 in 500 males, most are not detected until later childhood. The outward markers of small testicles and long limbs are rarely noticed early in life. Spermatogenesis is always impaired and infertility is usual.

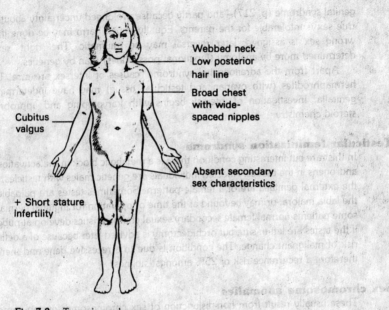

Webbed neck
Low posterior
hair line

Broad chest
with wide-
spaced nipples

Cubitus
valgus

Absent secondary
sex characteristics

+ Short stature
Infertility

Fig. 7.2. Turner's syndrome.

Late and early puberty

Girls reach puberty on average a year before boys and achieve their growth spurt 2 years earlier (p. 25). The age of puberty is influenced by genetic as well as environmental factors; when there are problems, it is important to enquire about the age of the parents' puberty.

Children (especially boys) and their parents frequently seek advice about 'late puberty'. However, absence of any signs of puberty at the age of 14 in girls and 16 in boys does not necessarily require investigation especially if there is a family tendency to late puberty. The measurement of height is useful, for physiological delay is more probable in short boys. However, for short girls who have delayed puberty it is important to exclude Turner's syndrome. The vast majority of children with 'late' puberty are perfectly normal: they need reassurance, moral support and patience. Exceptionally there is pituitary or gonadal insufficiency.

Much less often the doctor is consulted about early (precocious) puberty. True precocious puberty includes spermatogenesis or oogenesis, and is rare. It results from premature secretion of gonadotrophins. Slightly less rare is precocious pseudopuberty, in which secondary sexual characteristics develop abnormally early, but there is no growth of the gonads and no gametogenesis. The isolated precocious development of breasts (mammarche or thelarche), periods (menarche) or pubic hair (pubarche or adrenarche) is less rare. Precocious puberty occurs more frequently in girls than in boys, and in Blacks than in Whites; in the majority of instances the cause is unknown. A wide variety of intracranial disturbances, including tumours, hydrocephalus, meningitis and encephalitis, may lead to pubertal changes. Tumours arising in the adrenals or gonads may also cause precocious pseudopuberty. Boys with the adrenogenital syndrome will develop precocious pseudopuberty if left untreated.

Gynaecomastia in adolescent boys is almost always physiological and self-limiting. This does not prevent it being a considerable social embarrassment.

FURTHER READING

Buckler JMH. *The Adolescent Years*. Castlemead Publications.

Chapter 8
The Child with Learning Problems

A child's education is the equivalent of an adult's occupation and is second only to his family life in the influence it has upon his future. Indeed, children who get little or no support or encouragement at home may find more sympathy and understanding at school. It is therefore of great importance that:

1 children are in the best possible state of health—physical, mental and emotional—to benefit from their educational opportunities from the very beginning;

2 the educational system offers a sound basic curriculum with a wide variety of additional options in an environment which encourages learning and builds on success;

3 children leave school self-confident, healthy, and with career/job aspirations appropriate to their interests and to their educational achievements (which may not coincide with their parents' ambitions).

The educational system in the UK is a 'mixed economy' of state-run and privately run schools running side by side. The pattern of education they offer will meet the needs of about four-fifths of all children. The remaining one-fifth, for a variety of reasons listed below, will need either some modification of the educational programme in mainstream schools or, if the problems are more severe, education in a special school designed, staffed and organized to meet their needs.

The main medical problems which can affect children's education may conveniently be considered in groups, but there is a degree of overlap, and not infrequently children have problems in more than one group.

1 Physical—motor

This group includes disorders such as cerebral palsy, spina bifida and muscular dystrophy (see Chapter 9) and severe congenital abnormalities, especially of the limbs. Children with restricted mobility may not be able to join in games and physical education or to climb stairs. They need extra time to negotiate long corridors and may need handrails. Wheelchairs cannot negotiate stairs and need wide toilets. Problems of manipulation may prevent the use of normal writing implements: special pens or an electric typewriter may be needed.

2 Physical—sensory

Impaired vision or hearing present obvious barriers to education. If they are severe, and especially if they are combined (the deaf/blind), special equipment and specially trained treachers are necessary.

Mental

Children with moderately impaired intelligence are usually best served by the provision of extra help in the classroom (usually non-teaching aides) in main-stream schools. More severe impairment often needs the facilities and specially trained staff of a special school.

Emotional

Emotional problems often reflect social problems at home. A few children are difficult to motivate, in sharp contrast to the normally insatiable appetite for information in young children. Rather more are hyperactive, aggressive, destructive or antisocial. Not only are they difficult to teach; they disrupt the classroom and make the teacher's task wellnigh impossible.

Communication

Some conditions already mentioned are likely to interfere with communication: deafness, for example, on the receptive side and the dysarthria of some forms of cerebral palsy on the expressive side. In addition, a wide variety of poorly understood disorders, including autism (p. 132) and dyslexia (p. 102), may cause severe difficulties. The detailed diagnosis of these problems, and the devising of a suitable educational programme, call for very special skills.

Chronic illness

Chronic illness can interfere with education in a number of ways. Intractable asthma may result in frequent absences from school with resultant poor academic progress. Epilepsy may place a few restrictions on physical activities. Diabetes and coeliac disease may affect meals taken at school. Chronic juvenile arthritis may limit physical activities.

MENTAL HANDICAP

Intelligence is a difficult thing to define, but it has to do with understanding, reasoning and the association of ideas. It is not closely related to memory or creativity, both of which may be evident to an astonishing degree in mentally handicapped people. Nor has it much to do with sociability, which may be conspicuous by its absence in the super-intelligent.

Intelligence can be measured by a wide variety of 'intelligence tests', the results of which are often expressed as intelligence quotients (IQ). The concept of a global IQ which reveals all we need to know about a child's learning ability has given way to more detailed testing of the several components of intelligence. This provides a more comprehensive picture of the particular strengths and weaknesses of the individual child, and hence an indication of the particular kinds of help he needs at school.

It is important that children with special educational needs are identified, and their needs determined, well in advance of school age. The 1981 Education Act requires that local education authorities are notified of such children not later than their second birthday so that appropriate steps can be taken.

Aetiology

If global IQ is measured in an unselected population, the distribution curve is approximately Gaussian, with a longer tail to the left (low IQ) than to the right. Most people with IQs between 2 and 3 SDs below the mean are part of the normal distribution curve, and often have parents of low IQ. Most children with still lower IQs have some organic cause for their mental handicap, congenital or acquired:

1 75% are congenital abnormalities resulting from:
(a) chromosome abnormalities (30%), e.g. Down's syndrome;
(b) metabolic disease (under 5%), usually recessively inherited, e.g. galactosaemia, phenylketonuria;
(c) neurocutaneous syndromes (under 5%), often dominantly inherited, e.g. tuberose sclerosis, neurofibromatosis;
(d) other genetic causes, e.g. X-linked mental handicap and some cases of microcephaly;
(e) idiopathic (40%)—the cause cannot be identified.
2 25% are acquired. The brain may be damaged:
(a) prenatally, e.g. alcohol abuse, infections (rubella, CMV);
(b) perinatally, especially in very premature babies, by haemorrhage, hypoxia, meningitis, septicaemia, hyperbilirubinaemia, hypoglycaemia;
(c) postnatally by trauma (including non-accidental injury) or infection (meningitis, encephalitis).

Developmental delay

One of the main reasons for recommending that all young children should undergo regular developmental assessment (p. 39) is to detect any significant delay as early as possible. Another reason is to reassure parents who are unnecessarily anxious about their child's development. Mental handicap is likely to present as delayed development, unless there are physical features (e.g. Down's syndrome, microcephaly) which permit prediction of handicap before it is evident. It is, however, important to appreciate that although all mentally handicapped children are late developers, the reverse is not necessarily true. If the results of developmental tests are to be expressed numerically, they are expressed as a developmental quotient (DQ) rather than an IQ until intelligence can be adequately tested. In practice it is much simpler and more useful to express a child's achievement in a particular field or ability as appropriate to the average child of a particular age (e.g. his head control is at the 3-month level).

Faced with a child who is reported or found to be late smiling, sitting, walking or talking, the following points need attention:

1 If the delay is not gross, is there anything in the history which might explain the delay? Was the baby very premature? Has he spent long periods in hospital? Has he had proper care at home?
2 Is he delayed in all developmental fields or only in selected aspects? A mentally handicapped child will be retarded in all areas, although gross motor development may be better than social and language development. A child whose development is normal in any area is unlikely to be mentally handicapped.

3   Can a specific cause be found for a specific delay? If speech is delayed, is he deaf? If walking is delayed, has he muscular dystrophy?

4   A single assessment, especially if the child is having an 'off' day, may be an inadequate basis for decision-making. Although delay in recognizing, for example, deafness, is to be avoided, it is equally important not to express anxieties or initiate investigations prematurely. Re-examination, when progress can be assessed, is often helpful.

5   Although progressive (degenerative) brain disease is rare, it is important to establish that the skill in question was never achieved, rather than achieved and later lost.

Differential diagnosis

There are three stages in the diagnosis of a 'late developer':

1   Is the delay significant or does the child fall within the range of normal? This requires experience, but some charts (e.g. Denver developmental scale p. 40) provide a normal *range*.

2   If significant, what is the nature of the problem—mental handicap, deafness, social deprivation?

3   If there is mental handicap, what is the cause? This may be relevant to treatment and useful for genetic counselling. Investigation will include biochemical screening of blood and urine for metabolic disorders, serological tests for prenatal infections, neuroradiological studies and EEG.

Management

A few causes of mental handicap are preventable. Genetic counselling may prevent recurrence of autosomal recessive disorders; rubella immunization should be universal; babies are screened at birth for phenylketonuria and hypothyroidism (and, in some centres, for rarer metabolic disorders); improvements in perinatal and neonatal care should help. Secondary prevention is possible for conditions which can be diagnosed prenatally, although even for Down's syndrome this has made relatively little impact.

For the great majority of mentally handicapped children, their condition is incurable, the cause is often unknown, and the more carefully they are looked after, the longer they live. These circumstances place great strains on their families. Handicapped children can take up all the time and energies of both parents, leading to physical exhaustion (especially as the children get older and heavier), neglect of siblings and the breakdown of marriages. The problems are multiplied in single parent families.

The principles of management are to help the child to develop to his full potential, however little this may be, and to offer all possible help and support to the family. Many mentally handicapped children have additional problems such as cerebral palsy, epilepsy or deafness. Full assessment is therefore essential before any treatment programme is drawn up. Although the health services have an important role in helping children with cerebral palsy, epilepsy and other associated problems, it is the social and educational services which have the chief responsibilities for helping mentally handicapped children and their families. Many systems have been devised for encouraging maximal progress. Some are variations on traditional methods which have been properly assessed. Some, which unfortunately attract great media attention, play (to their considerable profit) on the eternal hope of parents that a cure may be found. Doctors must be understanding of parents who decide to try unorthodox methods, and must be prepared to help pick up the pieces if disappointment follows.

The main forms of family support available are:

1 Home visits by an individual who can become a friend and offer a shoulder to cry on, but is at the same time well informed about practicalities.

2 Provision of equipment for use at home, from incontinence pads to bath hoists, and adaptations to the home such as ramps for wheelchair access, or downstairs toilets.

3 Respite care, whereby the handicapped child periodically goes to stay with a foster family or into residential care.

4 Financial assistance such as Attendance Allowance, Mobility Allowance or help from the Family Fund.

Dental care is particularly important for the mentally handicapped. Some dentists specialize in their care.

Down's syndrome

This affects approximately 1 in every 600 babies; is less frequent for younger parents and more frequent for those over 35 years. Most children with Down's syndrome have an extra chromosome 21 resulting from non-disjunction at the time of gamete formation. A few result from translocation (interchange) or other abnormality involving chromosome 21. Parents who are translocation carriers are at substantital risk of having further affected children.

Prenatal diagnosis is possible by culturing fetal cells obtained by amnio-centesis or chorion villus sampling. Usually these tests are offered only to older couples and are not always taken up, so have made little impression on the birth prevalence of the condition. Non-invasive tests involving biochemical parameters (including *low* maternal serum AFP) and possibly ultrasound scanning are being developed.

Although none of the characteristic features of Down's syndrome is patho-gnomonic, and any may be present in a normal child, the association of several features usually enables a clinical diagnosis to be made (Fig. 8.1). Recognition in very small preterm babies is more difficult, and the condition is easily overlooked in aborted fetuses:

1 The skull is brachycephalic: both face and occiput are flattened. At birth a 3rd fontanelle may be present, just anterior to the posterior fontanelle.

2 The palpebral fissures are slightly oblique with prominent epicanthic folds (hence the old term 'mongol'). Tiny pale spots (Brushfield spots) appear on the iris as it becomes pigmented, forming a concentric ring around the pupil. The eyelashes are sparse. Squint, cataract and nystagmus are common.

3 The mouth is small and drooping. After infancy the tongue becomes large and furrowed and often protrudes. The pinna may be an abnormal shape.

4 The neck is short and broad with excess skin posteriorly.

5 The hands and fingers are short. A single transverse palmar crease (simian crease) is common, as is a short, incurved little finger (clinodactyly). There is

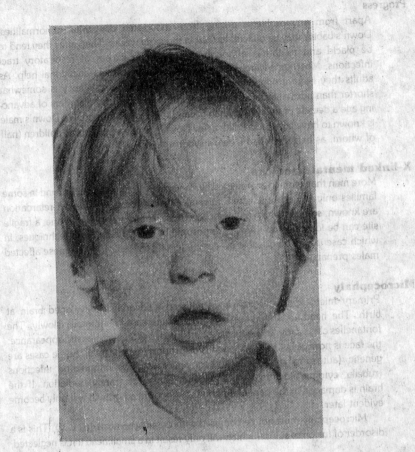

Fig. 8.1 A 5-year-old with Down's syndrome.

often a wide gap between the first and second toes, with a longitudinal plantar crease running from that gap.

6   There is hypotonicity and hyperextensibility.

7   Development is delayed in all aspects, although early gross motor development may be almost normal.

8   Associated congenital abnormalities are common, particularly congenital heart disease (especially VSD and AV canal) and duodenal atresia or stenosis.

Diagnosis

This can usually be made with confidence on clinical grounds but should be confirmed by chromosome analysis, which is also necessary for genetic counselling.

Progress

Apart from any problems arising from associated congenital abnormalities, Down's babies may be difficult to feed in the early weeks. Thereafter they tend to be placid and to thrive, although they have an excess of respiratory tract infections. Most are severely retarded and require special educational help. As adults they require continuing supervision. Their life expectancy is somewhat shorter than normal because they develop the degenerative disorders of advancing age a decade or two earlier than usual. Libido is diminished. No Down's male is known to have fathered a child: a few Down's females have borne children (half of whom, as expected, had Down's syndrome).

X-linked mental handicap

More men than women are affected by non-specific mental handicap, and in some families only males are affected. Several different forms of X-linked retardation are known, some of which are associated with macro-orchidism. In one, a fragile site can be identified on the X chromosome by special laboratory techniques, in which case it may be possible to identify female carriers or to diagnose affected males prenatally.

Microcephaly

Primary microcephaly is associated with an inadequately developed brain at birth. The head circumference is small and increases abnormally slowly. The fontanelles close early. In severe cases, the infant has a characteristic appearance: the face is normal but the skull vault is disproportionately small. Some cases are genetic (autosomal recessive). Others are caused by intrauterine infections (rubella, cytomegalovirus), toxins (alcohol abuse) or (rarely) radiation. If the brain is damaged in the perinatal period, the poor head growth will only become evident later.

Microcephaly must not be confused with craniosynostosis (p. 120). This is a disorder of fusion of sutures which will only result in a small head if it is neglected.

DISORDERS OF SPEECH AND LANGUAGE

Normal speech development is described on p. 47. Medical advice may be sought about children who are late in beginning to talk, or whose speech is thought to be abnormal. Most of these children are, in fact, normal. Some children have a sizeable vocabulary before their first birthday while others say little until 3 or 4 years old. A lisp is a common phase of speech development. Many 3 and 4-year-olds trip over their words because their thoughts and questions tumble out of their minds more quickly than they can articulate them. The average 4-year-old asks 26 questions an hour!

Nevertheless it is important not to overlook a significant cause of delayed or abnormal speech. Furthermore, it is often helpful to refer any child with a speech problem to a speech therapist so that parents can be advised how best to help. The wrong kind of parental intervention can make the problem worse.

If speech development is delayed:

1 Is the child being spoken to? Speech is learned by imitation.
2 Can the child hear? Deafness is an important cause of speech delay (p. 104).

Less commonly, the hearing mechanism is intact but the brain cannot interpret the sounds heard.

3 Are other fields of development delayed? If so, mental handicap must be considered (p. 95).

4 Is there evidence of emotional/behavioural disorder? Late speech is usual in autism (p. 132).

There is a strong link between language delay and later educational difficulties. A child with delayed speech should therefore be assessed as early and as expertly as possible.

The main abnormalities of speech are disorders of fluency (stammer/stutter) and of articulation. Stammering is common in young children and is much more common in boys than in girls. It usually goes spontaneously, especially if it is ignored. If it persists into school age it becomes a barrier to communication and a social embarrassment. Speech therapy is helpful in preventing it from becoming permanent.

Articulation disorders include:

1 Consonant substitution (e.g. 'Come' is pronounced 'Tum'). A few substitutions are normal in young children acquiring speech skills, but occasionally they persist, or are so numerous as to make the child unintelligible to others.

2 Nasality, resulting from cleft palate, including the submucous variety (p. 162), or nasopharyngeal incompetence.

3 True dysarthria, as in some kinds of cerebral palsy (p. 117).

4 Faulty enunciation, in which bad example, orthodontic problems or a wayward tongue may play a part.

Nasal escape may need surgical correction, but speech therapy is the principal form of help for all these problems.

SCHOOL DIFFICULTIES

There are many reasons for poor performance at school:

1 Social/Cultural. Parents who do not cooperate with the school and who do not encourage school attendance and school work.

2 Neurological/Psychological. Though major mental handicap will usually have been detected before school age other disabilities of hearing, vision, fine motor skills, perception, and learning may not.

3 Chronic ill health (e.g. asthma). It is important to check that the illnesses do warrant school absence.

4 School refusal (phobia) by an emotionally disturbed child, or truancy by older children whose parents are usually unaware of the school absence until notified by the teacher, social worker or police.

If a healthy child of normal intelligence and good vision and hearing has educational difficulties, an emotional problem will often be found. There may be unhappiness at home, or at school (from bullying or fear of a teacher), or parental over-expectation or indifference. Conversely, emotional problems may be the result of learning problems. A report from the school is an important part of the assessment of the schoolchild. More detailed assessment of intelligence and abilities by an educational psychologist will provide recommendations for remedial help.

When a child's reading ability is more than 2 years behind that whic
expected for his *age*, he is said to have reading backwardness. This is a comm
condition of boys and girls, particularly in those from social classes IV and V,
in children with an overt neurological disorder or a mild neurodevelopme
fault. A smaller group of children are said to have *specific reading retardati*
their reading age is more than 2 years behind their *mental age* (as measured
IQ testing). They are much worse at reading, speech and language than at ot
skills, and are particularly recalcitrant to treatment. This is commoner in boys
occurs in all social classes. It is not associated with neurological abnormalit
Some of these children are said to suffer from '*dyslexia*', but the term is fall
out of favour because of early inaccurate descriptions of it. All types of read
problems are commoner in large families, and all children with them need skil
assessment and help.

Severe *clumsiness* is another important cause of school difficulties. Ap
from difficulty with dressing or physical activities, some clumsy children n
have great difficulty with writing and drawing. They may be considered wron
to be stupid or lazy. Their incoordination may represent a mild form of cereb
palsy. Whatever the cause, once the problem is recognized the children can
taught to overcome many of their difficulties.

Special educational needs

The normal educational provision of mainstream schools meets the needs
about 80% of children. The remaining 20% need something more or somethi
different. In the past, some of these children were labelled according to the natu
of their problem (e.g. mental handicap, physical handicap, deaf) and were plac
in special schools bearing similar labels. The rest tended to flounder in the botto
layer of mainstream schools, often leaving without any educational qualificatior

More recent policy (in the UK) rests on three principles:

1 The earliest possible recognition or anticipation of special educatior
problems.

2 The detailed assessment of the child's needs through psychological, medic
social, parental and other reports.

3 The integration of children with special problems into mainstream school
unless their educational needs would be better met in the setting of a speci
school.

There is a statutory duty to inform the education authorities, at the earlie
opportunity, of any child who may have special needs. Education for suc
children may start as early as 2 years and such early education is particular
important for children with visual or hearing impairment who need to establis
good methods of communication with teachers and other children before form
education is possible. All children with special needs undergo a comprehensiv
assessment which results in a report ('Statement') which is discussed with th
parents and then forwarded to the education authorities who have the respons
bility for the child's educational provisions and any further assessment. Th
process of assessment is sometimes referred to as 'statementing'.

VISUAL IMPAIRMENT

Severe visual impairment is a terrible handicap at any age. When it is congenital, or even when its origin is in the pre-school years, it presents a serious threat to satisfactory development and education.

Local authorities keep a register of children with severe visual problems so that the families can be helped and suitable education planned. Experienced home advisers from either the local authority or the RNIB (Royal National Institute for the Blind—a charitable organization) visit the family to provide continuing advice and support. They provide practical advice e.g. 'Wear noisy shoes and give a running commentary about all your household activities so that he can understand and learn about the things he hears, sometimes smells and feels, but never sees'. Severe visual impairment requires formal education by methods not involving the use of sight; the specialist schools for the blind teach braille. For children with sufficient sight to use educational material involving large print and type, there are residential school for the 'partially sighted'. Both types of school are few in number, and the child is almost certain to be resident in one some distance from home.

Squint (strabismus)

Nearly 1 in 15 children have a squint when they commence school. The incidence is even greater in children with brain damage or mental handicap.

Babies sometimes falsely give the impression of having a squint because of a low nasal bridge, epicanthic folds, or wide-spaced eyes (hypertelorism). This is a pseudo-squint and unimportant. But a true squint is always abnormal. Methods of testing for a squint are given on p. 31.

Any child with a squint should be referred to an eye specialist who will exclude the rare but serious causes for a squint which include cataract, glaucoma, retinal disease and retinoblastoma, and then organize a plan of management. An untreated squint may cause the child to adopt an unusual tilt of the head or other posture to improve binocular vision in certain directions. More seriously, a young child suppresses the information from the defective eye in order to avoid blurred images and double vision. Unused, the eye becomes 'lazy' and can develop permanent amblyopia (diminished acuity of central vision). Treatment before the age of 6 should always prevent this. After the age of 10 a 'lazy eye' is likely to remain useless for life. A common treatment for young children, which is as unpopular with them as it is with their parents, is for the good eye to be occluded with a patch in order to force the child to use the lazy eye. This is often done for a period of several months before spectacles or other treatment is offered. With patience and determination children over the age of 2 years can be persuaded to keep patches or spectacles on most of the time.

For many young children with a squint resulting from poor visual acuity, early use of spectacles is sufficient treatment in itself. Severe squints, particularly if paralytic, may require surgery—if only for cosmetic reasons. After operation orthoptic exercises may be organized to encourage the child to stimulate binocular function.

HEARING IMPAIRMENT

Hearing exists before birth and can be demonstrated in neonates. They startle to a loud noise, or become quiet in response to a diminuendo growl. Some neonatal units use an auditory response cradle to screen the hearing of the newborn. An infant's hearing is most easily tested at 7–8 months of age when the child has an insatiable curiosity for new sounds. All children should be tested at this age using the tests described on p. 46. Appropriate tests are available for toddlers. Pure tone audiometry is not usually possible before 3–4 years. In younger children, auditory evoked responses are necessary for accurate diagnosis.

Deafness may originate from pre-, peri- or postnatal factors:

1 Prenatal factors include hereditary deafness, maternal infection (e.g. rubella) and malformations of the ear. Congenital rubella deafness is sometimes progressive and may not be detectable for months or years.

2 Perinatal factors include cerebral hypoxia and kernicterus.

3 Postnatal factors include meningitis, encephalitis, otitis media, and ototoxic drugs.

Congenitally deaf babies babble normally for about 6 months but then become quieter, do not talk but communicate by gesture. They may also have temper tantrums or other behavioural problems.

Most deaf children have some residual hearing, and so will be helped by a hearing aid which can be fitted as early as 3 months of age. That is the start of the treatment, not the end. The child requires prolonged exposure to speech and sounds at a level that he can hear with the hearing aid.

Skilled help is needed from a team of otologist, audiologist, hearing-aid technician and specially trained teachers. Education for the deaf can be started from 2 years, but most deaf children will enter the partially hearing unit of a nursery school at 3–4 years and then progress to similar units attached to normal schools or to special schools for the deaf. A few children behave as if deaf but respond to hearing tests normally. Theirs is a problem of auditory discrimination, an inability to interpret sounds.

FURTHER READING

Hall DM. *The Child with a Handicap.* Blackwell Scientific Publications.
Illingworth RS. *The Development of the Infant and Young Child.* Churchill Livingstone.

Chapter 9
Neuromuscular Disorders

Brain growth and development occur early in life. Neurone formation is completed within 3 months of conception. Half the increase in head circumference between birth and adult life occurs in the first 1.5 years. Myelination is largely complete by the age of 3 years, and the establishment of dendritic connections by 5. The brain is particularly vulnerable in this early period. Its normal development can be disturbed by a wide variety of factors:

1 Genetic:
    (a) single gene defects (e.g. tuberose sclerosis);
    (b) chromosome aberrations (e.g. Down's syndrome).
2 Prenatal:
    (a) drugs (e.g. alcohol abuse);
    (b) infections (e.g. rubella).
3 Perinatal:
    (a) extreme prematurity;
    (b) metabolic disturbances (e.g. hypoxia).
4 Postnatal:
    (a) infections (e.g. meningitis);
    (b) trauma (e.g. road accidents).

Brain damage may be manifest as seizures (fits), cerebral palsy, mental handicap or other disorders of learning (Chapter 8) or behaviour (Chapter 10). Progressive, degenerative brain disorders are rare. The spinal cord may be affected by congenital abnormality (e.g. spina bifida), infection or trauma. Peripheral neuropathy is extremely rare in children.

SEIZURES

A seizure is the result of an abnormal paroxysmal discharge by cerebral neurones. The terms seizure, fit and convulsion are interchangeable, but the public often associates convulsions with fever (benign) and fits with epilepsy (worrying). Fits are common in childhood: 6% of children have had a fit by the age of 11 years. The pattern and prognosis varies with age (Fig. 9.1).

Neonatal seizures

Seizures are common in the first month as a result of birth injury, metabolic and infective causes or developmental abnormalities (further details are given on p. 78).

Infantile spasms

Infantile spasms are a rare and serious form of seizure characteristically commencing between the ages of 1 month and 6 months. The infant doubles up,

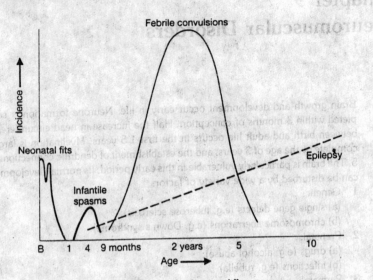

Fig. 9.1. The incidence and type of seizure at different ages.

flexing at the waist and neck, and flinging the arms forward—a 'salaam' spasm; less commonly it is an extensor spasm. Associated mental subnormality is common. The EEG usually shows a characteristically disorganized picture—hypsarrhythmia. Corticosteroids may suppress the fits. The final outcome is related to the cause, which may be metabolic or structural but often no cause is found. A previously suggested link with whooping-cough vaccine appears ill-founded.

3   Febrile convulsions

Four per cent of pre-school children have had a seizure. By far the commonest is a febrile convulsion, which is defined as a seizure occurring between 3 months and 5 years of age associated with fever but without evidence of intracranial infection or defined cause. Although they may be recurrent they should be distinguished from epilepsy (which is characterized by recurrent non-febrile seizures). A family history of febrile seizures is often present.

The seizures are generalized with clonic movements usually lasting less than 10 minutes. They are precipitated by a febrile illness rather than by fever itself and tend to occur at the start of the illness. Upper respiratory tract infections are the commonest association. The CNS is normal and there are no neurological signs once the seizure has ceased. Half the children will have further febrile convulsions with future illnesses, but very few have seizures after the age of 6. Prolonged, focal or frequent seizures, or an EEG which is abnormal more than 2 weeks after the seizure, suggest a diagnosis of epilepsy.

Seizures are frightening to the family and it is common for the parents to think their child is dying. In addition to reassurance, immediate therapy consists of the following:

1 Laying the child semi-prone with the neck slightly extended so that secretions drain out of the mouth and do not obstruct the airway.

2 Cooling the child. Paracetamol is helpful. Excess clothing or bedclothes should be removed. Occasional sponging with tepid water (which does not cause skin vasoconstriction) is needed.

3 Antibiotics, if an infection such as otitis media is present.

The main problem for the doctor is in deciding whether to admit the child to hospital. If there is any suspicion of meningitis, lumbar puncture is mandatory. If there is clear evidence of an associated infection, home treatment is reasonable, particularly if there is a history of previous febrile convulsions, but meningitis can complicate otitis media and pneumonia and is easily missed once antibiotics have been started.

Long-term management consists of explaining to the parents the relatively benign nature of febrile seizures and teaching them how to recognize and manage future seizures, how to use antipyretic agents safely and effectively, first aid for a seizure, and when and how to seek emergency assistance. Long-term prophylactic anticonvulsant therapy is occasionally used for selected children with recurrent febrile convulsions.

4 Epilepsy

A seizure in a previously healthy child is only exceptionally due to a metabolic disturbance (e.g. hypoglycaemia) or to organic brain disease. Careful clinical examination and appropriate investigation are therefore essential. However, the usual reason is idiopathic epilepsy (recurrent non-febrile seizures of unknown cause). About 1 in 200 schoolchildren are affected. The fits may be generalized or partial and take a wide variety of forms in children: in between attacks the child is perfectly well. It is exceptional for the doctor to have an opportunity to witness a fit and the diagnosis rests principally on the history, with help sometimes from the EEG which is consistently abnormal in 60%. Diagnosis can be difficult (see p. 109) and it is important not to attach the label 'epileptic' to a child without good reason. It may be difficult to remove.

Generalized seizures

Grand mal

Major epileptic attacks classically comprise a tonic phase (continuous muscle spasm) which may start with a cry and, if prolonged, lead to cyanosis: then a clonic phase (jerking) which may be associated with tongue-biting and frothing at the mouth; then relaxation, unconsciousness and a period of drowsiness and/or confusion. Children often sleep after an attack. Indeed, any recurrent symptom or symptom-complex in a child which is regularly followed by sleep is likely to be an epileptic phenomenon. Attacks may occur when the child is tired or over-excited, but often for no apparent reason. Intermittent photic stimulation (a standard activating procedure used when EEGs are recorded) triggers fits in some children, usually when they are watching a malfunctioning TV screen or sitting very close to the TV. The EEG may show bilateral, slow-wave, subcortical seizure discharges. Major fits can last any time from less than a minute to over an hour (status epilepticus). Prolonged fits can, by causing hypoxia, lead to brain damage, especially in the temporal lobes.

First aid for a major attack consists of lying the child semi-prone, with the head to one side to allow drainage of secretions; loosening tight clothing around the neck so that the airway is clear; and gentle restraint to prevent the child injuring himself. The fit can be stopped by anticonvulsant drugs given intravenously, intramuscularly or rectally.

Prophylactic therapy lies in regular medication, usually until the child has been fit-free for at least 2 years. Useful drugs for grand mal include carbamazepine, sodium valproate, phenytoin and phenobarbitone (p. 226). The prognosis is good for children who are otherwise healthy, have a normal EEG and respond promptly to preventive therapy; less good for those with mental handicap or cerebral palsy, with persistent seizure activity on EEG, and in whom a variety of drugs, alone or in combination, fail to give adequate control.

Most children with epilepsy attend normal school; only a tiny minority have such intractable epilepsy that special schooling is required. It is important that the teachers know how to recognize and deal with any seizure. Although the child should take part in most activities he may need extra supervision for swimming, and it may be wise to prevent him from doing activities such as high diving, rope or rock climbing and canoeing. Some doctors forbid cycling in traffic if the child has had a seizure in the previous 2 years, though seizures are uncommon during any concentrated activity.

Status epilepticus refers to the state in which a person convulses or has a series of convulsions for over 60 minutes without recovering consciousness in between. Apart from external injury hypoxic brain damage may result. Therefore all fits must be stopped fast. Intravenous diazepam is the drug of choice in hospital. This is combined with securing an adequate airway, administering oxygen, protecting the child from injury and, over a longer period, maintaining fluid and electrolyte balance. At home, intramuscular paraldehyde or rectal clonazepam are most effective.

Petit mal

Petit mal is uncommon; the onset is always in childhood. It is not caused by organic brain damage and the intelligence and behaviour of the child are normal. An attack consists of a very brief absence of awareness lasting less than 5 seconds and accompanied by blinking. The eyes may roll up. The child does not fall down. He may present with school difficulties because of 'day dreaming' or inattention.

Petit mal can be provoked by encouraging the child to hyperventilate hard for 2 minutes. The characteristic EEG shows a 3 per second spike and wave pattern. Ethosuximide and sodium valproate are the most effective drugs (p. 226).

Partial seizures (focal epilepsy)

The seizure discharge is confined to a focus of neurones and does not become generalized. Sometimes the focus is at the site of previous cerebral damage (for example, some children with temporal lobe epilepsy have acquired it as a result of anoxic damage to the temporal lobe during prolonged convulsions). Carbamazepine is a particularly effective treatment. The most important types are given below.

Temporal lobe

Temporal lobe lesions are the cause of complex partial seizures (*psychomotor epilepsy*). They are more common than petit mal, and may present as motor, sensory or emotional phenomena singly or in combination. Any convulsive movements are less repetitive than Jacksonian seizures. The diagnosis is confirmed by EEG. The children, especially boys, may have psychiatric and behavioural problems and, occasionally, impaired intelligence.

Jacksonian (minor motor seizures)

These are simple partial seizures which may occur without any disturbance of consciousness. The convulsive movement predominantly affects one area of the body only, though the clinical manifestations may 'march' to involve the corner of the mouth and the peri-ocular muscles. Sometimes the seizure is followed by temporary weakness of an involved limb (*Todd's paralysis*). Jacksonian fits in children have a less serious prognosis than in adults.

General management of epilepsy

Although most seizures are idiopathic it is important to search for a primary cause from a careful history and examination, for fits can be caused by space-occupying lesions, meningitis, hypoglycaemia, hypertension, and many other causes. A rare but interesting group are children with neurocutaneous syndromes in which a skin lesion is associated with an intracranial lesion. Many of these are genetically determined and associated with mental handicap. It is important to examine carefully the child's skin for the pathognomonic skin lesion.
Sturge–Weber syndrome: port wine stain (p. 185).
Neurofibriomatosis: café-au-lait spots.
Tuberose sclerosis (epiloia): depigmented and pigmented areas, particularly on the trunk and, later on, papules over the nose and face (adenoma sebaceum).

The principles of anticonvulsant therapy are to use the lowest dose of the safest drug that suppresses fits and to continue the drug until at least 2 years after the last fit. In addition to the drugs already mentioned, nitrazepam and clonazepam may be useful. The advent of modern anticonvulsant drugs has reduced greatly the number of children with intractable epilepsy who require treatment with a ketogenic diet, or with neurosurgery. Measurement of drug levels in plasma may be useful to check adequacy of dose and patient compliance.

Conditions simulating epilepsy

In toddlers, *breath-holding attacks* (p. 132) and *masturbation* may mimic fits. In the latter case the child's legs are extended and crossed and may either be held stiff or move rhythmically. The face is flushed, there are often grunting noises, and the child protests if an adult interferes.

In young schoolchildren, *benign paroxysmal vertigo* is an occasional cause of confusion. The child becomes giddy and frightened, clings onto an adult, and may vomit or show nystagmus. Night terrors (p. 131) may also occur at this age.

In older schoolchildren, especially girls, fainting (syncope) is common. It most often happens in school assembly or in church, following an abrupt change

Table 9.1. Main features differentiating a seizure from a faint (syncope).

	Seizure	Faint
Age	Any	8–15 years
Timing	Day or night	Day
Situation	Commonly during inactivity	Standing
Prodrome	Brief (twitching, hallucinations, automatisms)	Long (dizziness, sweats, nausea)
Duration	Variable	Under 5 minutes
Tonic–clonic movement	Common	Rare
Colour change	May be cyanosis	Pallor
Injury, e.g. tongue-biting	Common	Rare
Incontinence of urine	Common	Rare
Epilogue	Drowsiness, confusion or headache. Rarely partial paralysis	Quick full recovery. Never paralysis

from sitting to standing. The child feels giddy, becomes pale and falls if not caught. There is no twitching: recovery is spontaneous and rapid (Table 9.1).

Episodic *behavioural disorders* may cause diagnostic difficulty, and many children with psychological problems are wrongly thought to be epileptic. Nocturnal episodes may be especially difficult to interpret. Continuous 24-hour EEG recordings can be helpful.

Similarly, 24-hour ECG recordings may reveal the cause of sudden loss of consciousness, especially if the episodes are related to exercise (p. 146).

ACUTE INFANTILE HEMIPLEGIA

Acute infantile hemiplegia presents as a seizure and is a rare but serious condition. A previously healthy young child has severe convulsions, usually unilateral, becomes comatose and develops hemiplegia. A vascular cause can sometimes be demonstrated. Recovery is slow and usually incomplete: there is residual weakness affecting especially the hand, and a visual field defect is common. Epilepsy, impaired intelligence and/or behavioural disorders follow in at least half the children.

MENINGITIS

This is essentially a disease of childhood—80% of all cases occur in the first 5 years of life. The younger the child, the more difficult is diagnosis and hence the greater is the risk of residual brain damage. The importance of considering the *possibility* of meningitis in any sick child cannot be over-emphasized. In infants, a delay of only hours in diagnosis can make the difference between complete and incomplete recovery. If there is *any* doubt about the possibility of meningitis, a diagnostic lumbar puncture is mandatory.

The early symptoms are often non-specific: fever, irritability or drowsiness and vomiting. Fits are common and may be preceded by more localized twitchings. An older child will complain of headache, photophobia and possibly neck- or backache.

In children past infancy, the classic signs of meningeal irritation may be present. Neck stiffness—a reluctance to flex the neck—may be demonstrated by encouraging the child to look at his feet or kiss his knee. Head retraction is a sign of advanced meningitis. Kernig's sign is often present, but its absence does not exclude meningitis.

In infants these signs are less dependable but the anterior fontanelle is at first 'full' (a slight increase in tension) and later bulging. They may have a high-pitched, piercing cry. Meningitis may arise as a complication of middle-ear infection so the eardrums must be carefully examined (see also Meningism, p. 113).

Common viral causes of meningitis (aseptic meningitis) are mumps and echoviruses. Mumps meningitis often occurs in the absence of other manifestations of mumps and is especially common in boys. The only common complication is unilateral deafness. Mumps meningitis is a rare sequel to mumps vaccination. Poliomyelitis (p. 113), once a common and serious form of aseptic meningitis, is hardly ever seen in countries that provide mass immunization against the disease. Bacterial (purulent) meningitis is slightly less common than viral but is more serious and more likely to cause brain injury. In neonates, meningitis may be caused by a wide variety of different micro-organisms, Escherichia coli being the commonest. In childhood, the three main pathogens are Neisseria meningitidis (Gram-negative diplococcus), Haemophilus influenzae (Gram-negative bacillus) and Streptococcus pneumoniae (Gram-positive diplococcus).

Meningococcal meningitis develops with frightening rapidity and there may be evidence of meningococcaemia (p. 112). Pneumococcal and H.influenzae meningitis develop more gradually, sometimes as a complication of upper or lower respiratory tract infection.

Investigation

Prompt lumbar puncture is imperative. Papilloedema is not a contraindication, provided only 1–2 ml of CSF are removed. Gram stain and differential cell count provide the most useful immediate information. Usually it is possible to differentiate an aseptic meningitis from a purulent meningitis from the CSF examination as shown in Table 9.2 provided the child has not received recent antibiotics.

Table 9.2. Characteristics of CSF.

	Normal	Viral meningitis	Bacterial meningitis
Appearance	Clear	Clear or hazy	Cloudy or purulent
Cells/mm³	0–4	20–1000	1000–5000
Type	Lymphocytes	Lymphocytes	Polymorphs
Protein g/l	0.2–0.4	0.2–1.0	0.4–10
Glucose mmol/l	3–6	3–6	0.5–6

When the findings are equivocal it is usual to treat as if there is a bacterial pathogen. Faeces, CSF and throat swabs can be cultured for viruses, and in all cases blood culture should be performed. The ESR may be of help in meningitis, for a value of over 50 (or an equivalent plasma viscosity) makes a viral aetiology most improbable. Tuberculous meningitis (p. 235) may present as a lymphocytic meningitis.

Treatment

Children with bacterial meningitis are treated initially with intravenous antibiotics. Until the bacterium has been identified chloramphenicol and ampicillin may be used. This is combined with whatever supportive and symptomatic therapy may be needed—anticonvulsants, analgesics, or intravenous fluids for a collapsed child. Improvement should occur within 36 hours, and early treatment is usually associated with complete recovery though pneumococcal meningitis tends to follow a slower course. Slow recovery or relapse may be a sign of persisting infection or of a subdural effusion. Aspiration and drainage of the effusion is needed.

Meningococcal septicaemia (meningococcaemia)

This may occur with or without associated meningitis. It is a serious and frightening condition which is endemic in the UK. Small epidemics sometimes occur, though the infectivity within households is low. Pre-school children are most severely affected. The onset is abrupt and the course may be catastrophically fulminating with death occurring within 12 hours. The pathognomonic sign is a purpuric rash, which may be sparse or so profuse that the lesions coalesce to form large ecchymoses. One mode of death is from peripheral circulatory failure associated with haemorrhage into the adrenal glands (Waterhouse–Friederichsen syndrome). An intravenous infusion should be set up on any child suspected of having menigococcal septicaemia: antibiotics are given intravenously, and the line can be used for plasma expanders or hydrocortisone in the event of collapse. Household contacts should be given a 2-day course of rifampicin or ciprofloxacin (as should the affected child before leaving hospital).

Outcome

Meningitis is a serious condition. Some children die and a proportion, especially infants, incur permanent brain damage resulting in mental handicap, cerebral palsy, deafness, hydrocephalus or epilepsy. Viral meningitis is treated symptomatically and has a lower incidence of complications. Recurrent meningitis is most rare, and should provoke a close search for a dermal sinus. This is a small pit found in the midline of the back which provides a portal through which micro-organisms reach the meninges.

Encephalitis

Encephalitis is an illness in which cerebral symptoms (e.g. fits and drowsiness) or neurological signs are not accompanied by definite signs of meningitis. The CSF usually has raised protein and/or lymphocytes. The commonest form in childhood is acute disseminated encephalomyelitis associated with infection (also called meningoencephalitis or post-infectious encephalitis). It is not caused by direct infective invasion of the brain, and usually occurs about a week after one of the common infectious fevers—measles, rubella, chicken pox or mumps. Most cases are mild, but occasionally severe and permanent brain damage ensues as a result of demyelination. Encephalitis very rarely follows immunizing procedures (pertussis, measles); the risk is about 10 times smaller than that associated with the corresponding infection.

Meningism

This is the term given to the symptoms and signs, particularly the neck stiffness, that may be present at the time of an extracranial infection. It may be associated with otitis media, tonsillitis, cervical adenitis, arthritis of the cervical spine or pneumonia. Often a lumbar puncture has to be done to ensure that the CSF is normal and the child has not got meningitis.

Anterior poliomyelitis

Once known as infantile paralysis (although unusual in infants) or simply 'polio', this potentially crippling disease has been almost totally eradicated from developed countries by immunization but remains common in deprived communities elsewhere. The virus spreads from (and to) the upper respiratory tract, but exerts its devastating effects on the anterior horn cells of the spinal cord and the brain stem (polio-encephalitis). Paralysis is of sudden onset and associated with muscle tenderness and malaise, is maximal at the start and variable in extent but usually asymmetrical. The signs are those of a lower motor neurone lesion without sensory loss. Recovery is usually incomplete. If the respiratory muscles are involved, artificial ventilation is needed to sustain life. Immunization confers virtually complete protection.

Acute infectious polyneuritis

This is an uncommon condition chiefly affecting children aged 2–10. It is characterized by degeneration of the peripheral nerves and nerve roots. The cause is unknown though it tends to occur shortly after various acute infections. There is an ascending paralysis which in the space of a few days progresses to a symmetrical peripheral neuritis with motor loss, sensory loss and absent tendon reflexes. Provided that the child can be nursed through the acute stage complete recovery gradually occurs.

The CSF is either normal or shows a high protein but normal cell count (Guillain–Barré syndrome).

HYDROCEPHALUS

Hydrocephalus arises from obstruction of the normal CSF circulation either as a result of congenital abnormality, e.g. aqueduct stenosis (Fig. 9.2) or from postnatal causes such as meningitis, intracranial haemorrhage or tumour. It is commonly associated with spina bifida.

In congenital hydrocephalus the size of the head at birth varies from normal to gross enlargement. As the CSF accumulates under pressure the head enlarges rapidly, the skull sutures separate, the anterior fontanelle bulges and the scalp

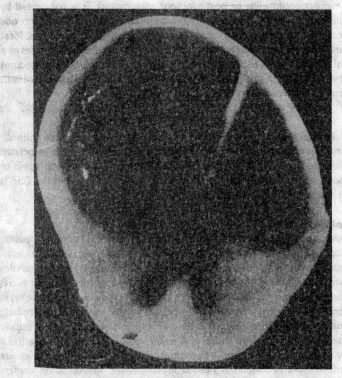

Fig. 9.2. CT scan showing extensive hydrocephalus, involving mainly the occipital lobes, as a result of aqueduct stenosis.

veins appear prominent. The eyes turn downward (setting sun sign). In the older child whose skull sutures are united, obstruction to CSF pathways causes headache, vomiting and other symptoms of raised intracranial pressure. It is the *rate* of skull expansion rather than any single measurement that distinguishes the infant with hydrocephalus from the normal infant with a big head (Fig. 9.3). (See p. 29 for method of head measurement.)

Untreated hydrocephalus may lead to permanent brain injury, so prompt surgical treatment is often needed. The usual practice is to bypass the obstruction by inserting a Spitz–Holter or a Pudenz valve. This is a one-way valve connected to two catheters, one of which is inserted into the lateral ventricle whilst the other is passed via the internal jugular vein into the right atrium or into the peritoneal cavity (Fig. 9.4). Depending on the cause of the obstruction and the speed of treatment, normal brain development and function is possible. Low grade infection and other technical problems often prevent the valves from being as permanently effective as desired.

Not every child with a big head has hydrocephalus. The differential diagnosis includes familial megalencephaly (measure the parents' heads), hydranencephaly (the skull is full of fluid and transilluminates in a dark room) and achondroplasia

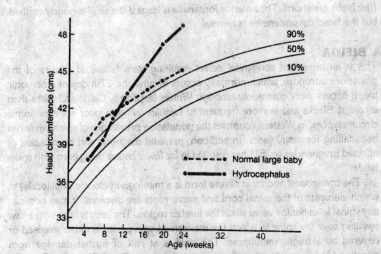

Fig. 9.3. The head circumference of a normal large baby increases at a rate parallel to the centile lines; that of the hydrocephalic increases at an abnormal rate.

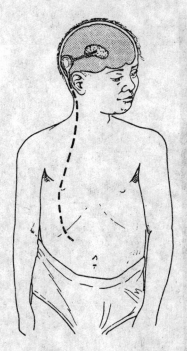

Fig. 9.4. Pudenz valve draining CSF from the lateral ventricle into the peritoneal cavity.

(the limbs are short). The anterior fontanelle is large if the skull is poorly ossified, but the head circumference is normal.

SPINA BIFIDA

This is an important congenital defect resulting from failure of closure of the posterior neuropore, which normally occurs around the 27th day of embryonic life. It occurs more commonly amongst Whites (especially Celts) and Sikhs than amongst Blacks and is more frequent in families living in poor socioeconomic circumstances. In Western countries the population prevalence of spina bifida has been falling for many years. In addition, prenatal diagnosis and termination of affected pregnancies (p. 51) has resulted in far fewer babies being born with spina bifida.

The commonest and most severe form is a *meningomyelocele* (myelocele) in which elements of the spinal cord and nerve roots are involved. It may occur at any spinal level but the usual site is the lumbar region. The baby is born with a raw swelling over the spine in which the malformed spinal cord is either exposed or covered by a fragile membrane. The cord is at risk of further damage from infection, drying out or other direct physical trauma (Fig. 9.5).

The majority are associated with hydrocephalus, particularly as a result of the Arnold–Chiari malformation in which a tongue of malformed medulla and

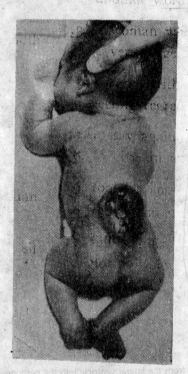

Fig. 9.5. Meningomyelocele, shortly after birth.

cerebellum protrudes down through the foramen magnum, preventing free escape of CSF from the 4th ventricle.

The main physical problems from meningomyelocele are:

1 Legs—partial or complete paralysis below the level of the lesion, with associated sensory loss. Secondary hip dislocation and leg deformities occur, especially talipes (club foot).

2 Head—associated hydrocephalus with possible brain damage.

3 Bladder—neuropathic bladder with overflow incontinence and recurrent urinary tract infections leading to kidney damage.

4 Paralysis of the anus if the relevant spinal cord segments or roots are involved, resulting in faecal incontinence.

The emotional and social problems for the child and family are massive, varying from the frequent hospital admissions and attendances to the problems of providing suitable education for a paraplegic, incontinent child.

Surgical treatment is not advised if the baby has gross nydrocephalus, kyphosis, severe paralysis or associated major congenital anomalies because these indicate a very poor prognosis. Any baby with spina bifida needs early expert assessment, and surgical closure when appropriate. This will protect the cord from further damage. Subsequently, the child may be helped by treatment of associated hydrocephalus. Orthopaedic procedures may improve function, especially of the hip. A variety of calipers and walking aids may improve mobility, but most children need wheelchairs. Intermittent or continuous catheter drainage of the bladder may allow continence and prevent kidney damage, but sometimes urinary tract surgery is also needed. The therapeutic programme is therefore formidable, and the majority are still handicapped at the end.

Meningocele

This is less common and less serious. The sac of CSF is covered by meninges and skin and contains no neural tissue. Cosmetic surgery is not urgent.

Encephalocele

Encephaloceles are protrusions of brain through the skull, covered by skin, usually in the occipital region. If large, they are likely to be associated with severe brain abnormality.

Spina bifida occulta

Spinal X-rays of young children often show an apparent defect of the neural arches of the lower lumbar vertebrae, but there is usually a cartilaginous bridge which calcifies later. True spina bifida occulta is rarely associated with any neurological problem, although if there is an external 'marker' in the lumbar region (hairy tuft, naevus, lipoma), intraspinal pathology is more probable.

CEREBRAL PALSY

Cerebral palsy is a disorder of posture and movement resulting from a non-progressive lesion of the developing brain. In general the term is rarely applied to brain lesions incurred after the age of 2 years. Children with cerebral palsy are sometimes called 'spastics', but not all have spasticity (see below). It occurs once in every 1500 live births.

The brain abnormality underlying cerebral palsy may result from genetic, prenatal, perinatal or postnatal factors, but often it cannot be determined. The basic pathology may be a developmental abnormality, pre- or postnatal brain infection; physical or chemical injury to the brain, or a vascular accident.

The presentation varies according to severity. In the most severe cases poor sucking or altered muscle tone may arouse suspicion soon after birth. More often cerebral palsy is first suspected within the subsequent few months when the child's motor development is delayed—there may be poor head control or lateness in sitting. It is important to realize that, although the brain lesion is fixed and non-progressive, the disorder it causes varies in the early years as different movement patterns are acquired or persist beyond their time. A hypotonic infant may become hypertonic during the first year of life.

Terminology

1 *Tone* is the resistance to passive movement. Increased tone may be of two kinds, spasticity or rigidity.

> (a) *Spasticity* arises from a lesion of the cortex or pyramidal tract pathways. The increase in tone is found in one direction only, e.g. supination of the forearm, not pronation; dorsiflexion of the wrist, not plantar flexion. Spasticity is often associated with increased reflexes and possibly with clonus.
>
> (b) *Rigidity* arises from a lesion of the basal ganglia or extrapyramidal pathways. The increase in tone is present in all directions and sometimes has a cogwheeling feel to it.

2 *Involuntary movements* (dyskinesia). These may be choreiform, athetoid or dystonic. The difference between them is sometimes quite subtle, the choreiform movements being of a more jerky nature than the sinuous athetoid movements. Dystonia tends to cause twisting movements involving part, or the whole, of the body.

3 *Ataxia*. This manifests itself as a tremor on intention, difficulty in walking heel-to-toe, nystagmus and dysarthria.

4 *Diplegia*. Predominant involvement of the legs, though the arms may also be affected.

5 *Quadriplegia*. Involvement of all four limbs.

6 *Hemiplegia*. Involvement of one arm and one leg on the same side.

Management

The management of these children is a difficult art. Early comprehensive assessment is essential because:

1 There is often other associated handicap, e.g. mental handicap, epilepsy, defects of vision and hearing.

2 Disordered posture and movement can lead to permanent deformities.

3 Cerebral palsy can present major problems of management at home and at school.

Therefore apart from a detailed history and general examination the following have to be assessed: vision, hearing and intelligence, and the emotional and social state of the child and home. The fact that the divorce rate of parents with cerebral palsied children is high is just one expression of the great stress which such children place on the family. It is a degree of stress that can be considerably reduced by an energetic and compassionate doctor. Early physiotherapy aims to establish a normal pattern of movement by facilitating normal postural reflexes and inhibiting the awkward persisting primitive reflexes, and to prevent deformity. Orthopaedic surgery can help to prevent and correct deformity in spastic cerebral palsy and neurosurgical intervention with posterior rhizotomies may reduce spasticity.

Attempts to help the child to speak may often need to be supplemented with other systems of communication, e.g. symbols, signing and computers.

Prognosis

This depends mainly on the presence or absence of associated handicaps, and in particular on the intelligence of the child. With normal intelligence, the problems of even the most severe motor handicaps may be overcome. The quality of the management itself affects the prognosis. A severely affected child may require education in a special school where expert physiotherapy, occupational therapy, teaching and other facilities are available.

Children less severely affected, including most with hemiplegia, manage at normal school, and the least severely affected of all do not always reach the specialist. Their clumsiness, their inability to march in step or their difficulty in copying shapes may make them an object of derision at school without it being realized that they are suffering from mild cerebral palsy.

SPACE-OCCUPYING LESIONS

These cause raised intracranial pressure as a result of their own size and by interfering with normal CSF drainage. Headache, misery and irritability are common early symptoms and are followed by unsteadiness, vomiting and visual disturbances. Fits may occur.

In infancy the anterior fontanelle is tense and the skull sutures widened. In young children, tapping the skull may yield a 'cracked pot sound'. In older children, papilloedema occurs early. Skull X-ray may show 'copper beaten' bones with widened sutures and erosion of posterior clinoids. In any child suspected of having a space-occupying lesion, CT brain scan must be carried out promptly. The most important space-occupying lesions are given below.

Neoplasm (p. 212)

Cerebral abscess

Focal infection in the brain arises from:
1 Extension from the middle ear;
2 Congenital cyanotic heart disease (especially Fallot's tetralogy);
3 Infected emboli from the lungs or elsewhere in the body.

There is a slow invasive stage during which the child is feverish, drowsy and complains of headache, followed a week or two later by dramatic features of raised intracranial pressure and focal neurological signs. The CSF at first shows a sterile leucocytosis and later a raised protein; the ESR is always elevated, but there is not always a blood leucocytosis. The commonest pathogens are streptococci or staphylococci. Early antibiotic treatment can lead to complete cure, but once formed and encapsulated the abscess may only subside after drainage.

3 Subdural haematoma

Bleeding into the subdural space is usually caused by trauma. Subdural haematomata are commonest under the age of 2, in contrast with cerebral abscesses which are uncommon in infancy. One important cause of subdural haematoma is non-accidental injury (p. 242). The symptoms may present acutely or chronically. The latter are more difficult to diagnose, for the traumatic episode may be several weeks past, and the infant may have relatively non-specific features of failure to thrive, low-grade fever and convulsions. Unless it is drained, the haematoma may enlarge as the blood breaks down and more fluid is absorbed into the sac. In this way signs of an expanding space-occupying lesion develop and permanent brain damage may occur. Neurosurgery is then urgently required.

CRANIOSYNOSTOSIS (craniostenosis)

Premature fusion of one or more of the skull sutures results in an unusual-shaped head and may compress the brain or cranial nerves. The prognosis depends upon which sutures are affected. Premature fusion of all sutures results in a bulging forehead, proptosis and brain compression which requires urgent surgery. Premature fusion of a single suture, usually the sagittal, causes a misshapen head which may require surgery for cosmetic reasons. The cause is unknown. Sometimes there is a hereditary factor, and frequently there are associated skeletal abnormalities. The diagnosis is confirmed by skull X-ray.

Skull asymmetry is common in early infancy, but the sutures and fontanelles are normal; one side of the forehead and occiput are displaced forward. The asymmetry becomes less with growth and does not cause problems. There may be associated chest asymmetry. The skull asymmetry is often referred to as plagiocephaly, but this term is more properly reserved for asymmetrical craniosynostosis.

PROGRESSIVE NEUROMUSCULAR DISORDERS

Among the most distressing disorders of childhood are those that strike previously healthy child and progress inexorably towards incapacity and death over months or, more often, years. They may affect principally the brain, the spinal cord or the muscles; many are genetically determined and few are open to effective treatment.

Progressive brain degeneration can result from several different conditions, many of which are due to autosomal recessive genes. They can be grouped into those that affect the grey matter (e.g. the lipidoses such as Tay–Sachs disease) and those that affect the white matter (leucodystrophies). They present with loss of previously acquired skills, usually in the first year or two of life; in general, the earlier the onset, the more rapid the progress. Precise diagnosis may be difficult but is important because treatment is available for a few of these conditions and genetic counselling is important.

Spinal muscular atrophies are a group of conditions due to autosomal recessive genes which present with progressive weakness affecting predominantly the lower half of the body. The infantile form of spinal muscular atrophy (Werdnig–Hoffmann disease) is evident in the early months of life and progresses to death within a year or so; forms with later onset progress more slowly. Those with onset in late childhood often enjoy a reasonably active adult life.

Myopathies (muscular dystrophies) are also variable in their age of onset, rate of progress and mode of inheritance.

Duchenne (pseudohypertrophic) muscular dystrophy

This is the commonest type of muscular dystrophy in childhood. It is due to an X-linked recessive gene and therefore only affects boys. The gene for the disorder and its related protein (dystrophin) have now been identified. The condition presents as late walking (over 18 months), with an abnormal waddling gait or with difficulty climbing stairs. There is often marked lumbar lordosis (Fig. 9.6). Affected boys develop enlargement of the calves due to fatty infiltration ('pseudo-hypertrophy') with absent knee jerks. If asked to stand from sitting on the floor, they often 'climb up their legs' (Gowers' sign) to compensate for the weakness of the hip and knee extensors. Affected boys lose the ability to walk at about the age

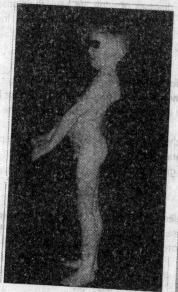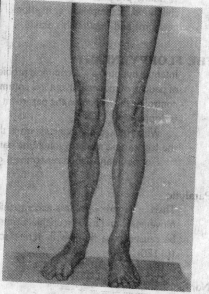

Fig. 9.6. The boy on the left has Duchenne dystrophy. There is pseudohypertrophy of the calves, marked lumbar lordosis and winging of the scapulae. On the right the wasted thighs and hypertrophy of the calves is seen in a boy with Becker dystrophy.

of 10 years and tend to die of pneumonia or myocardial involvement in their late teens or early twenties. A proportion have intellectual impairment. A grossly elevated serum creatine phosphokinase level is present from birth and most female carriers have a slightly raised level.

A milder form of pseudohyertrophic muscular dystrophy (Becker) is due to an allelomorphic gene on the X chromosome. Symptoms develop later and disability is mild. Limb girdle dystrophy (autosomal recessive) and facio–scapulo–humeral dystrophy (autosomal dominant) rarely present in childhood.

There is no cure for muscular dystrophy. Therapy is supportive and there should be active physiotherapy and mechanical supports to prevent contractures and deformity and to maintain mobility for as long as possible. Obesity is to be avoided. Because of the various forms of inheritance, a precise clinical and genetic diagnosis is important in order to provide reliable genetic counselling for the immediate family and other relatives. In some circumstances it is possible to identify carriers by genetic tests.

Other progressive disorders

Rett syndrome is an important cause of severe mental and physical handicap in girls. Although normal in early infancy, such girls begin to show evidence of slow psychomotor development towards the end of their first year. Subsequently they have unexplained loss of manipulative skills and speech associated with social withdrawal. Characteristic repetitive hand movements, e.g. hand wringing, rubbing or tapping is a feature of the inexorable decline.

Many progressive neuromuscular diseases of adult life have their onset in childhood. Examples are myotonic dystrophy (which may be lethal in the newborn) and Friedreich's ataxia.

THE FLOPPY INFANT

Infantile hypotonia is a common problem. Extreme examples are noticed because of paucity of movement, but it is commoner for it to present because of poor head control or the feeling on the part of an experienced mother or nurse that the baby is floppy.

When picked up under the arms the baby tends to slip from one's grasp and the feet can be made to touch the ears easily.

Floppy infants fall into two main groups as follows.

Paralytic

There is severe weakness accompanied by hypotonia. These infants make few movements and may be unable to raise their arm upwards against gravity. It can be caused by a number of rare disorders, including spinal muscular atrophy (p. 120).

Non-paralytic

More commonly there is hypotonia but only mild weakness. In these babies it is essential to search carefully for the primary condition causing the hypotonia. The possible causes include the following:

1   Severe mental handicap.

2   Cerebral palsy—many children who subsequently show spastic diplegia are floppy in early infancy.

3   Certain syndromes—Down's, Marfan's, osteogenesis imperfecta.

4   Benign congenital hypotonia. The hypotonia is present in the neonate and may be severe. It does not progress and after a period of several months slow improvement leads to complete recovery in most children. A few are found to have congenital myopathy (which has a characteristic muscle biopsy appearance), and they usually have mild muscle weakness.

5   Metabolic disorders—coeliac disease, rickets, glycogen storage disease.

Floppy infants present a difficult diagnostic problem. If no generalized primary cause is apparent, serum creatine phosphokinase, electromyography and muscle biopsy may be needed.

FURTHER READING

Brett EM *Paediatric Neurology*. Churchill Livingstone.

Dubowitz V. *The Floppy Infant*. Clinics in Developmental Medicine Ser.: Vol. 76: Spastics International Medical Publications.

Gordon N. *Paediatric Neurology for the Clinician*. Clinics in Developmental Medicine and Child Neurology, no 59/60. Heinemann.

O'Donohoe N. *Epilepsies of Childhood*. Butterworth.

Stark GD. *Spina Bifida*. Blackwell Scientific Publications.

Chapter 10
Emotional and Behavioural Problems

The requirements for normal physical and mental growth have been described in Chapter 1. This chapter is about the child's emotional growth, the things that may disturb it, and the ways in which this disturbance may present. At what age in childhood can one begin to talk about the emotions? Some newborn babies cry often, others are placid; there is no way of knowing whether their different behaviour indicates physical or emotional differences. Sudden loud noises or being dropped may elicit a 'startle' response in newborns, but one cannot tell whether they feel frightened. At 1–2 months the infant begins to become socially responsive, and if a smile is assumed to equate with a pleasurable sensation, one can begin to study emotional reactions.

Social responsiveness is a two-way process and in early life the mother is the vital partner. *Bonding* is the term used to describe the unique attachment that she develops for her child and which allows her to love, give to, understand and forgive her child. Outwardly it may be manifest by the way in which she holds her child, cuddles, kisses and fondles him, but the all important factor is the ability she has developed to cherish her child through good and bad times. Mothers do not necessarily love their baby at first, it may take several weeks, but it is important that in the early days after the birth parents have the chance to be alone with their baby in quiet, happy and untroubled surroundings.

Probably the most important requirement for healthy emotional development in the early years of life is constancy. The more widely used term, security, really only means that-which-makes-the-child-feel-secure, and leaves one wondering what it is. A close, personal and physical relationship with one person who provides food, warmth and comfort appears to be the earliest essential ingredient. Usually this will be mother, but on occasions it may be father, grandmother, foster-mother, or some other mother substitute. Initially the infant is aware only of mother, but as he grows he absorbs siblings, father and others into his world and begins to establish relationships with them. His horizons expand from mother to family to neighbourhood to school and beyond. At each stage there are new situations to explore, new relationships to establish. Each stage is built on the one before, which explains the crucial importance of the earliest stages.

Constancy implies that a person, and later a group, can be relied upon to provide the necessities of life, that the person or group is constantly available and does not change and that the responses to exploratory activities are constant. It follows that inconstancy arises when the child does not know to whom he should turn, when the composition of the group suddenly changes or he is suddenly removed from it and if he receives conflicting responses, for example, in terms of what he may or may not do. The rules themselves are not so important and will vary from one family to another; but everyone in the family needs to know the rules and to stick to them. In the early months and years the child is putting down his emotional roots. If the ground is forever being disturbed, the roots cannot grow.

The form that an emotional disturbance takes will depend in part upon the cause and in part upon the child's personality and the family patterns of response to stress. Disorders of eating and sleeping usually result from ill-judged or inconsistent handling by parents. Stress is likely to manifest itself as migraine if the child comes from a headache-prone family. The placid child is unlikely to have temper tantrums but may have recurrent abdominal pain. The toddler who feels challenged by the arrival of a new baby may resort to infantile behaviour.

In summary, the doctor is likely to be faced with two groups of children whose problems are basically emotional. The first comprises those with psychosomatic disorders, in which the emotional stress causes physical symptoms. The second comprises those with overt disorders of behaviour. Psychosis is rare.

STRESS AND ITS SYMPTOMS IN CHILDHOOD

Emotional stresses in children, as in adults, frequently manifest themselves in physical symptoms. Emotional disorder can occasionally be life-threatening, as in anorexia nervosa. Far more common are recurrent abdominal pains, headache, vomiting or limb pains as manifestations of stress. Habit spasms (tics), compulsive drinking and sleep disorders in older children are also usually due to psychological stresses.

The kinds of stress that may precipitate symptoms vary enormously, as does the severity of the stress. Some children are of a buoyant temperament and can ride almost any crisis; others are sensitive plants and bow before every emotional breeze. The following is by no means a comprehensive list but includes some of the stresses most commonly afflicting children.

1 *Acute separation.* The death of a parent or of a much-loved grandparent, emergency admission to hospital or moving house are examples of acute separations. These are most upsetting to young children around 2–4 years old who are conscious of the separation but unable to understand the reason.

2 *Parental discord.* All children are conscious of the relationship between their parents and will be aware of any deterioration. When discord develops, the child is likely to be involved and invited to take sides in the contest. This is a devastating experience for all but the most insensitive. A history of recent separation or divorce is not uncommon when children present with stress symptoms, but the symptoms have usually begun long before the break. Indeed, if the marriage is damaged beyond repair, a physical separation of the parents may provide the only foundation on which to rebuild the child's security.

3 *Inconsistent handling.* If a child is permitted something by one parent that is denied by the other, or forbidden by parents but encouraged by grandparents, or punished on one occasion and ignored on another, this is likely to encourage the more flamboyant kinds of behavioural disorder such as temper tantrums, breath-holding attacks and difficulties with eating and sleeping. The intelligent child is quick to play off one adult against another, or to achieve his own ends by alarming or distressing the adults around him. Diplomacy and blackmail can be learned from an early age.

4 *Boredom.* If children have time on their hands the effect varies with age. The infant who is deprived of companionship and playthings will be delayed in his development. Without encouragement and practice, motor skills, speech and social activities lag. The bored toddler who is confined to his cot 'to keep him out of mischief', having thrown all toys overboard, can choose between cot-rocking, head-banging, pulling out his hair (trichotillomania), masturbating or playing with his excreta. Older children who are bored may take to truancy and vandalism.

5 *Sibling rivalry.* Toddlers are expected to be jealous of their new baby brothers and sisters. In fact, most toddlers, and especially first-borns, delight in the new baby, but may resent the time that their mother devotes to it. If there is regression or aggression, it is likely to be directed against the mother rather than against the baby. When the new baby is old enough to be mobile and to interfere with the elder sibling's activities, jealousy will become more obvious. At school age, constant comparisons between siblings with different capabilities and interests can devastate the less clever or the clumsy. It is almost unbelievable how many parents will discuss their children in their presence, as if they were not there, drawing unfavourable comparisons with other children. This may lead to anti-social behaviour such as lying, stealing, truancy or wanton destruction.

6 *Great expectations.* Closely allied is the unfavourable comparison between the child's achievements at school and the expectations of his parents or teachers. Parents naturally want their child to do well but may form an unrealistic idea of his capabilities or set their hearts on a career for him which he could never achieve. Although many a child 'could do better if he tried', not everyone is destined for an honours degree. If parents constantly nag when he is doing his best, psychological breakdown will follow. Recurrent abdominal pain, if it leads to school avoidance, may be the presenting symptoms, or there may be more serious disturbance.

7 *Acute emotional shock.* Sometimes a child is witness to, or involved in, an acutely distressing situation—a road accident, a sudden death, or sexual abuse. Such an incident may lead to hysterical symptoms (e.g. mutism), to disturbed behaviour (e.g. night terrors), or to acute physical symptoms (e.g. over-breathing).

Periodic syndrome

Stress may manifest as recurrent abdominal pains, headaches, limb pains, vomiting or other symptoms. Many descriptive terms have been used—abdominal migraine, bilious attacks, acidosis, cyclical vomiting—and the term 'periodic syndrome' is used to include all recurrent symptoms or symptom-complexes attributable to stress. They are common.

Recurrent abdominal pain is by far the most common of these symptoms and it has usually persisted for a year or more by the time medical advice is sought. The pain is almost always central, does not radiate widely and may be associated with nausea. It can be severe, the child becoming quiet and pale. It occurs at any time of day, without obvious precipitating cause, but scarcely ever wakes the child at night. The child may complain of pain several times in a week and then not at all for a month or two. As children with recurrent abdominal pain are usually of school age, the parents often suspect some stress at school. The class teacher, whose report is often helpful, suspects some tension at home and is often right.

Careful clinical examination, including microscopy of the urine, supported if necessary by abdominal ultrasound scan, or barium meal, must be carried out to exclude organic causes of abdominal pain, and to provide a basis of reassurance for the parents. Constipation can cause pain, usually a pelvic discomfort relieved by defaecation. Rarely, abdominal pain may be the sole symptom of temporal lobe epilepsy. This would be suggested by a history of sleep following the pain, an abnormal EEG and a good response to anticonvulsants. Recurrent abdominal pain is sometimes the presenting symptom of coeliac disease or of food intolerance (especially milk).

Headache is a common stress symptom in children. It is usually frontal, sometimes vertical or occipital. It may be unilateral (migraine) and associated with nausea or vomiting, but a visual aura is much less common in children than in adults with migraine. In most cases, headache is the family stress symptom, and one or both parents will admit to migraine or sick headaches. Migraine sometimes results from sensitivity to food (chocolate, cheese) or food additives.

Vomiting is intimately connected with the emotions ('I'm sick of it all') but is less common than pain as a stress symptom. It occurs at a younger age than recurrent pains. As young children readily become ketotic and ketosis can cause vomiting, a vicious circle may develop.

After listening to the history, there are two useful supplementary questions. 'What sort of a boy/girl is he/she?' Children with stress symptoms are more often described as nervous, worriers, perfectionists or solitary than as placid, happy-go-lucky or gregarious. 'Who does he take after?' usually elicits a rueful smile and the admission that one or both parents are cast in the same die. This helps understanding. Examination reveals no disease, but bitten finger-nails may indicate the tension behind the smile.

It is not to be expected that stress symptoms will be spirited away, but much can be given by the exclusion of organic disease (especially the mythical grumbling appendix), by explanation of the nature of the symptoms and by encouragement not to pay undue attention to them. It is also wise for the doctor to make clear that he understands that the pains are real and not imaginary. Every effort should be made to identify stresses, and health visitors and teachers can be very helpful here, but often the symptom is being perpetuated by parental anxiety, in which case a careful history and examination coupled with firm reassurance may be all that is needed. Drugs should be avoided.

Enuresis

Enuresis is a common problem. The term is used to describe inappropriate voiding of urine at an age when control of micturition would be expected. Children learn to be dry by day at about 2 years, and by night at about 3 years. By 3.5 years, 75% of children are dry by day and night. Most children who wet have 'intermittent' enuresis; it is exceedingly rare to encounter children of school age with true 'primary' enuresis (i.e. who have never had a dry night). 'Secondary' or late onset enuresis refers to the situation when a child who has been dry for at least 1 year starts wetting again. Bed wetting (nocturnal enuresis) is a commoner problem than daytime wetting (diurnal enuresis).

Nocturnal enuresis

At 5 years, 15% of children wet their beds, by 10 years the figure is down to 5% and at 15 years 1%. *Noctural enuresis* is commoner in boys and in lower social classes. Its origins are multiple, and in any child may result from several factors. A genetic predisposition, with a positive family history, is common. Developmental delay may be a factor; just as some children are late walking so some are late at learning to control micturition. Stressful events at the time when the child was learning to get dry may interfere with the learning process and severe stress later in childhood sometimes causes a relapse of enuresis. Most enuretic children do not suffer from either a psychological illness or an organic illness.

Any condition causing polyuria (e.g. diabetes or renal insufficiency) or bladder irritation (e.g. urine infection) may cause bed wetting, but it is rare for bed wetting to be the *presenting* symptom of those illnesses. However, the child with enuresis should have a full physical examination, if only to reassure the parents who may be convinced that a disease is the cause. If as is usual the child has had a few nights completely dry, one can be sure that there is no defect in the mechanics of the urinary tract such as ectopic ureter or neuropathic bladder. The urine should be tested for glucose, and for infection.

Management of the enuretic child is a rewarding art. It is a condition that will go, and in most cases an enthusiastic doctor can accelerate the natural cure. Concern and time to listen and explain are vital. Sometimes the home situation, with the mother spending the days washing the sheets and the nights changing them, is so tense that the general atmosphere of stress and bad temper increases the wetting. Explaining to the parents that 1 in 8 of other 5-year-old children also wet the bed will help, and the child will be comforted to learn that at least three others in his class wet their beds. Punishment has little place; most children are anxious, indeed over-anxious to stop wetting. Rewards and encouragement may help. The child can be given a notebook, diary or chart in which to stick coloured stars after a dry night. This chart also helps the doctor assess progress. If the child micturates frequently during the day (has a small functional bladder capacity) he can be trained to hold on for longer to get the bladder used to a larger urine volume. Conditioning therapy by enuresis alarm is useful for children over the age of 7, and has a high success rate. There are two main types of alarm both of which depend upon the passage of urine completing an electrical circuit which sounds an alarm. The child then has to get out of bed, switch off the alarm and go to the toilet. The 'pad and bell' comprises a plastic mat, imprinted with an electrical circuit, on which the child lies, which is connected by wire to an alarm placed out of reach of the child. The 'body worn alarm' uses a tiny electrical sensor attached to the child's pants connected to a mini-alarm pinned to the pyjama jacket. Such alarms need to be used for 3 or 4 months and require much effort by the child and family, but at the end most children either awaken before they wet (and go to the lavatory), or sleep through without wetting.

Drugs have limited use in the treatment of nocturnal enuresis. Although both the tricyclic antidepressant drugs (e.g. imipramine) and antidiuretics (e.g. desmopressin) reduce bed wetting whilst the drug is being taken, most of those children relapse when the drug is stopped.

Diurnal enuresis (daytime wetting)

Of healthy children over the age of 5, 1% have troublesome daytime wetting. Two-thirds of them are reliably dry at night. The problem is commoner in girls and is usually the result of urge incontinence. (Urodynamic investigation would show bladder instability). Half the girls who wet by day have recurrent bacteriuria—the bacteriuria contributes to bladder instability and urge incontinence which itself results in damp, smelly pants which predispose to infection. There is an increased incidence of emotional disorder compared with children who merely wet the bed. With increase in age there is a natural tendency to become dry and that acquisition of dryness is accelerated by eradication of bacteriuria and an energetic management regimen which places responsibility on the child voiding more frequently and completely. In schoolboys daytime wetting tends to be associated with soiling and more overt behavioural disturbance.

Disturbance of bowel habit

Potty training may be started any time in the first 2 years, and a few parents choose to defer it for longer. If started very young, it is the parents who are training themselves to put a pot under the baby when he is going to pass faeces or urine, most commonly after a feed. This helps to establish a conditioned reflex, reinforced by praise when something arrives in the pot but not by punishing the reverse. Toddlers should not be left sitting on their pots for long periods, nor should potty-training be obsessional or coercive ('You can't until . . .', or, 'unless . . .'). Faulty bowel training predisposes towards constipation which may become life-long.

Disturbances of bowel habit in children comprise the following:

1 *Chronic constipation*, which may be complicated by faecal soiling.
2 *Faecal incontinence* resulting from neurological disorders (e.g. meningomyelocele).
3 *Encopresis*: deliberate defaecation in inappropriate places.
4 *Toddler diarrhoea* (p. 160).

Faecal soiling, which is most common at 5–10 years, begins as constipation leading to faecal retention. Sometimes this has been 'deliberate', starting during a negativistic phase of development and precipitated by coercive bowel training. Sometimes a hard stool has caused an anal fissure, an acutely painful condition which inhibits defaecation and increases constipation. At other times inadequate parental supervision has resulted in infrequent and incomplete bowel actions. The rectum becomes distended with impacted faeces right down to the anal margin. In extreme cases, only liquid matter can escape, causing spurious diarrhoea with faecal soiling, of which the child is unaware. His school companions, by contrast, are only too well aware of it, and the child with soiling may become a social outcast.

The abdomen contains hard, faecal masses, often filling the lower half of the abdomen. Rectal examination reveals faeces right down to the anus. There is unlikely to be confusion with Hirschsprung's disease which usually presents at a much earlier age and in which obstruction is only exceptionally as low as the anus. Unless there is diagnostic doubt, a barium enema is best avoided.

Management involves first the thorough emptying of accumulated faeces by enemata; suppositories are rarely adequate. Bowel training must then be instituted by regular toileting and the use of faecal softening agents such as disodium sulphosuccinate. Laxatives are often needed initially. The addition of fibre (e.g. bran) to the diet is helpful; ideally the whole family should adopt a high fibre diet. Instant success is not to be expected because the rectum takes time to resume its normal calibre and sensation. Admission to hospital is helpful if home management fails.

Encopresis is a symptom of serious psychological upset and the advice of a child psychiatrist should be sought.

Habit spasms (tics)

Repetitive, involuntary movements, involving particularly the head and neck, may occur in response to emotional stress. Tics are not rhythmical and cannot be stopped voluntarily. They are most frequent in boys aged 8–11 years. There may have been a reason for the movement initially—a twist of the neck in an uncomfortable collar, a forceful blink because of eyelid irritation—but the movement persists when the reason has gone. Entreaties (or threats) to the child to desist only serve to make it worse and the family are advised to try and overlook the child's irritating habit.

Sleep disorders

Sleepless children demoralize parents. Young children are demanding by day, but parents survive if they can enjoy peaceful nights. Sleeplessness may begin for a good reason, but persist as a bad habit. Children differ in their personalities from birth; some seem to be born 'difficult', while others are placid.

Young infants sleep most of the time and crying usually indicates hunger, thirst, cold or pain. It is difficult to be sure of the emotional needs for sound sleep at this age, but the infants of anxious or depressed mothers often seem to be tense and cry readily. A period of wakefulness during the day is common in early infancy (see 3-months colic, p. 83).

The most difficult sleep problems are usually seen in toddlers. Some do not settle down when put to bed; others sleep for a few hours and are then full of activity when the rest of the household is sound asleep. By the time advice is sought these habits have usually persisted for a long time and parents have tried both protracted and complicated bed-time routines, and the almost irreversible step of admitting the child to the parental bed. It is always noticeable that whilst the parents often look worn out, the offending child has boundless energy.

This problem can often be traced to one of two sources. It may date from an illness or upset in which a few broken nights were to be expected, but has been protracted by over-solicitous attention. The other common cause is putting the child to bed too early or at no fixed time. Children vary enormously in their sleep requirements and sometimes seem to need less than their parents. If put to bed early, either because they are thought to need so many hours' sleep or because parents like a little time together in the evening, they are wide awake and resent being confined to a cot.

Sleep problems are best prevented by a sensible routine and a firm line when unreasonable demands are made. Before resorting to drugs it is worth trying simple remedies. If the child is fearful of the dark, a night light or open door to a lit landing may bring calm. If the child demands the presence of mother until asleep, he may accept instead an article of her clothing as a talisman. If bad habits are firmly established, temporary use of hyponotics may be unavoidable. High doses are often needed initially. The right dose (as of any drug) is that which achieves the desired effect.

Nightmares are common at all ages. Parents, having experienced them themselves, are not usually very worried by them. They know that nightmares occur in normal people and that they do not mean major emotional upset. Measures such as leaving the bedroom door open, or a light on, may comfort the child who is frightened of going to bed. Nightmares occur during rapid eye movement (REM) sleep and are the culmination of a dream adventure, the details of which the child can remember immediately afterwards.

Night terrors are not common, but are most alarming. They occur mainly in the first hour or two of sleep. The child shrieks, sits up and stares wide-eyed and terrified as if being attacked by something only he can see. He may stumble out of bed and seem oblivious to the parents' soothing words. However, within a few minutes he will be sound asleep again and will remember nothing in the morning. The parents can be reassured that night terrors do not indicate serious psychological abnormality, that the child does not remember them, and that the child will outgrow them.

Night terrors occur during non-REM sleep, and occur abruptly (not as the result of a dream sequence). They are accompanied by an alarming rise of the pulse and violent respirations which may at times make the parents or doctor suspect an epileptic fit.

Sleep-walking may occur independently or as an extension of night terrors, though the sleep-walker tends to be slightly older (in the 6–12 year old range). The child gets out of bed and may walk around the house or even into the street. Although difficult to awaken, he can be guided back to bed. Regardless of that he will usually find his own way back to bed and to sleep. Although both night terrors and sleep-walking occur commonly the night after a stressful day, they should not be viewed as evidence of major emotional disturbance. Both conditions tend to be familial and to disappear before adolescence.

Crying babies

All normal babies cry. Excessive crying, especially at night, exhausts parents and invites physical abuse. Physical causes (e.g. earache) may be responsible for short-term crying. Persistent crying more often reflects household tensions. Mothers who seek advice about excessive crying are often afraid that they or their husbands will lose their tempers and damage the baby. The problem may sound trivial to a busy doctor but must *always* be taken seriously. The health visitor can often help.

Breath-holding attacks

Breath-holding attacks are common but harmless: they occur in 1–2% of children up to 3 years, and are precipitated by frustration or physical hurt. After one lusty yell the child holds his breath, goes red in the face, and may later become cyanosed and briefly lose consciousness. He then starts breathing again and is soon back to normal. Sometimes cerebral hypoxia is sufficient to cause brief generalized twitching, and the possibility of epilepsy may then be raised. A careful history will usually resolve any doubts. The attacks are benign and self-limiting. The parents require explanation and reassurance. If they can ignore the attacks, this is ideal. If they feel compelled to action, a little cold water over the head will relieve the tension all round. Sedatives and tranquillizers are not necessary.

The disorders so far described in this chapter lie within the competence of the general practitioner and paediatrician. Help from psychiatrists, psychologists and psychiatric social workers is usually needed to deal with antisocial behaviour in adolescents and with the more serious behavioural disorders that follow.

Severe behavioural disorders

Anorexia nervosa

This is uncommon in children, but important. It occurs more commonly in girls than in boys, and rarely before early puberty. In contrast to children who eat poorly because they are depressed, children with anorexia nervosa appear to have an abundance of energy strangely at variance with their microscopic food intake and steadily falling weight. They look ill but insist that they feel well. It is a serious disease which can be fatal, and requires hospital treatment under the supervision of a child psychiatrist.

Autistic behaviour

This incorporates certain characteristics of which the most constant are an avoidance of human contact (especially visual contact), delayed and restricted speech and an obsession with sameness—the same things, the same way, the same ritual. Autistic children prefer things to people and avoid your gaze. Sometimes the onset of symptoms is very early: a mother may say, 'As a baby he would never let me cuddle him.' This sort of behaviour is not uncommon amongst children with mental handicap, deafness, or blindness.

Infantile autism is autistic behaviour in children without other disability. Such children are often difficult to handle and always difficult to teach because of their inability to communicate. An undue proportion of them come from professional homes, and sometimes one or other parent shows mild autistic features—a preference for solitude, an unwillingesss to look you in the eye.

Hyperkinetic behaviour

In some ways this is a contrast to autistic behaviour. Children vary greatly in the extent of their spontaneous activities and it is impossible to define the limit between physiological and pathological degrees of over-activity. Many normal children are 'always on the go', 'never still', and need relatively few hours of sleep. Beyond this is the hyperkinetic syndrome in which these features reach an unreasonable degree. Hyperkinetic children are bursting with restless energy from dawn to dusk, and often much of the night as well. They move their attention from one thing to another in rapid succession and cannot be persuaded to concentrate on anything for more than a few seconds. They are easily distracted and seem incapable of sustained attention. In children of school age this presents a grave educational problem.

The hyperkinetic syndrome is more common in boys and in children with evidence of brain damage (mental handicap or epilepsy) which further complicates their education. Behaviour modification therapy can help. Methylphenidate may have a quietening effect while phenobarbitone paradoxically often makes things worse. In some children hyperactivity is caused or aggravated by particular foods or (more often) food additives such as artificial colourings. A properly supervised exclusion diet is worth trying: any improvement in behaviour will be evident within a few days.

FURTHER READING

Connell H. *Essentials of Child Psychiatry*. Blackwell Scientific Publications.
Graham P. *Child Psychiatry: a Developmental Approach*. Oxford Medical Publications.
Illingworth RS. *The Normal Child: Some Problems of Early Years and their Treatment*. Churchill Livingstone.
Jolly H. *The Book of Child Care*. Allen and Unwin.
Lask B and Fosson A. *Childhood Illness: The Psychosomatic Approach*. Wiley.

Chapter 11
The Cardiovascular System

INNOCENT MURMURS (also called benign, functional and physiological)
These occur in patients without any cardiac abnormality. They are often accentuated by fever, excitement and exercise, and disappear when the heart rate slows; they vary with respiration and posture. They are systolic or continuous. A diastolic murmur is never innocent. Three main types of systolic murmur are recognized.

Vibratory murmur—the character and pitch of the vibratory murmur are like the buzzing of a bee. It is very short and occurs in mid systole, but is less obvious when the patient sits up and extends his neck, and often disappears when he sits with his hands behind him and arches his back. It is commonest under the age of 10 years and usually disappears at puberty.

Pulmonary systolic murmur—the pulmonary systolic murmur is a soft, blowing ejection systolic murmur occupying the early part of systole, heard at the second left interspace close to the sternum and conducted upwards to the infraclavicular region. The differential diagnosis is a mild degree of pulmonary stenosis, but the second sound is normally split when the murmur is innocent, and the ECG and X-ray are *quite* normal. It is commonest in older children and adolescents.

Venous hum—a venous hum due to blood cascading into the great veins is a blowing continuous murmur best heard in the supraclavicular fossa, but often quite loud below the clavicles. The hum is abolished or greatly diminished when the internal jugular vein on the same side as the murmur is compressed, when the patient turns his head from the side to a midline position, and when he lies down flat.

CONGENITAL HEART DISEASE

In Britain, most heart disease in children is congenital. Eight out of every 1000 children born alive have a heart defect. There is a spectrum of severity in each defect from mild to severe and in every lesion changes take place as a child grows, sometimes for better and sometimes for worse. Most severe symptoms occur in the first year of life, particularly in the newborn infant, and urgent investigation and treatment are required. Mild lesions cause no symptoms, are compatible with a normal life and require no treatment. Nevertheless, children with severe lesions may have no symptoms yet treatment is necessary to prevent secondary changes in the myocardium, which will not reverse if surgery is delayed too long.

Primary myocardial disease and subacute endocarditis are rare. Rheumatic fever and rheumatic heart disease are still prevalent in developing countries but are rarely seen now in Britain.

Aetiology

In the majority of cases this is not known. Environmental factors play some part; maternal rubella in early pregnancy, the use of drugs such as thalidomide and phenytoin, maternal diabetes, alcoholism and smoking during pregnancy are all associated with an increased incidence of heart disease in the child. Congenital heart block is related to the presence of antibodies in the blood of mothers with connective tissue disease. In 5% of patients, chromosomal abnormalities are present, particularly Down's syndrome (atrioventricular defects), Turner's syndrome (coarctation of the aorta), 13 and 18 trisomy (septal defects). There are some rare autosomal dominant syndromes with cardiac abnormalities such as Marfan's syndrome (prolapsing mitral valves and aneurysm of the aorta) and Holt–Oram syndrome (septal defects). Atrial septal defects, hypertrophic obstructive cardiomyopathy and supravalvar aortic stenosis occur with a dominant form of inheritance with incomplete penetrance. Monozygotic twin individuals have twice the expected incidence of heart defects.

There is an increased incidence of complex heart disease in the Muslim Asian population, in whom the incidence of consanguinity is high.

In summary the most readily acceptable theory for the genetic basis of congenital heart disease is the multi-factorial hypothesis: there is a genetic susceptibility to develop congenital heart disease if the appropriate environmental hazard occurs.

Recurrence

The recurrence rate in siblings of patients with congenital heart disease is between 1 and 3% for the common lesions. Siblings usually have the same lesions. The risk to the offspring of a parent with congenital heart disease is greater and is in the region of 8%.

Classification

Eight lesions account for 85% of all congenital heart defects, and the remaining 15% is made up of combined complex and rare lesions.

Acyanotic

Left-to-right shunt: ventricular septal defect—incidence 30%

atrial septal defect—incidence 10%

patent ductus arteriosus—incidence 7%

Stenotic lesions: pulmonary stenosis—incidence 10%

aortic stenosis—incidence 7%

coarctation of the aorta—incidence 7%

Cyanotic

Tetralogy of Fallot—incidence 7%

Transposition of the great arteries—incidence 7%

Changes in circulation at birth

Before discussing the individual lesions it is worth recalling the changes that take place in the circulation at birth. These changes are relevent to congenital heart disease and explain why symptoms do not occur in some lesions until a few weeks after birth. In the fetus, only about 15% of the right ventricular blood enters the lungs, the rest passes through the ductus arteriosus to the descendng aorta; the ductus is as large as the aorta and pressures in the pulmonary artery and the aorta are equal. In the fetus there is a high pulmonary vascular resistance and the muscular pulmonary arteries are constricted and have a thick medial muscular layer.

After birth the following changes take place (Fig. 11.1):

1 The pulmonary vascular resistance falls and the pulmonary blood flow increases.

2 The systemic vascular resistance rises.

3 The patent ductus arteriosus closes.

4 The foramen ovale closes.

5 The ductus venosus closes.

There is dilatation of the lung vessels and normally the greatest fall in pulmonary artery pressure takes place in the first three days of life. While the ductus remains open there is preferential flow from the aorta to the lungs but the ductus closes functionally within 10–15 hours. It would be expected that in large communications between the two sides of the heart, such as patent ductus arteriosus and ventricular septal defect, the greatest left-to-right shunt would occur in the first

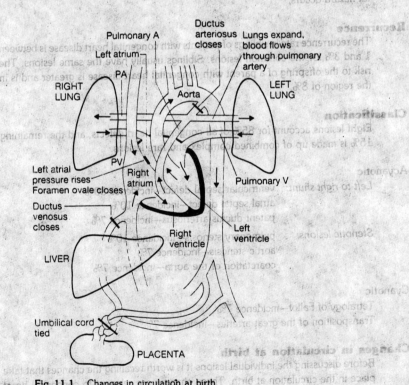

Fig. 11.1. Changes in circulation at birth.

three days. This does not in fact happen. The rate of fall of pulmonary vascular resistance proceeds more slowly and this helps the circulation to adapt more gradually and delays the onset of symptoms.

Pharmacological manipulation of the ductus

There are some heart lesions in the *newborn* infant which are incompatible with survival if the ductus arteriosus closes. These are pulmonary atresia, severe coarctation of the aorta and simple transposition of the great arteries without any septal defects. An intravenous infusion of prostaglandins will ensure the patency of the ductus and improve the baby's condition prior to surgery.

Conversely, in premature infants who require ventilation, it may not be possible to wean them off the ventilator because the ductus is widely patent. Indomethacin intravenously will result in closure of the ductus in some *premature* infants and surgery is avoided.

Diagnosis

Diagnosis can usually be made in the common lesions after clinical examination, chest X-ray and a 12-lead electrocardiogram. Nowadays the next investigation is an echocardiogram with Doppler echocardiogram when necessary. These are non-invasive tests and their use has resulted in a brisk fall in the number of diagnostic cardiac catheterizations and angiocardiography. As well as visualizing the various defects, gradients across valves can be measured and blood flows calculated. It is the best way of confirming a pericardial effusion and may also show vegetations associated with infective endocarditis.

LEFT-TO-RIGHT SHUNTS

Ventricular septal defect

The natural history is mainly related to the size of the defect, the changes that occur with growth, and the behaviour of the pulmonary circulation.

Small defects. Patients have no symptoms and the heart murmur is heard during routine examination. Of these 75% close in the first 10 years of life (the majority by 2 years) but closure goes on occurring in adult life. The only risk such patients run is of bacterial endocarditis.

Medium-sized defects. These cause symptoms in infancy. The increased pulmonary blood flow causes breathlessness, the child feeds slowly and weight gain is slow; heart failure may develop in the second or third months of life, often precipitated by a chest infection. Improvement occurs following medical treatment and as the child slowly gains weight, the defect becomes relatively smaller, symptoms lessen and further improvement occurs with the introduction of spoon feeding, but his weight lags behind normal. Chest infections are common and he is less active than his friends but by school age there is little difference from normal. Closure also occurs in these medium-sized defects and it is uncommon for pulmonary vascular disease to occur.

Large defects. Symptoms usually begin after the second or third week of life and heart failure occurs around 4–6 weeks of age, often precipitated by chest infection. It is difficult to control the heart failure by medical means, tube feeding is necessary and prolonged hospitalization is required. Following medical treatment one of the following changes may occur:

1 The patient improves, and as he gains weight the hole becomes relatively smaller, and surgery is not necessary. In 12% of these, the hole closes spontaneously. Both closure and reduction in size are commonly associated with the development of a thin mobile aneurysm of the membranous septum, which projects into the right ventricle and can be demonstrated on echocardiography.

2 Heart failure cannot be controlled and the child cannot feed independently. He does not gain weight and operation is necessary.

3 In about 10% infundibular stenosis develops. This is mild at first but gradually increases until a right-to-left shunt occurs and the lesion becomes a tetralogy of Fallot.

4 Aortic regurgitation occurs when the defect lies just below the aortic root; one of the valve cusps prolapses into the defect. It rarely occurs before 3 years but must be recognized as early as possible or the regurgitation will increase. Closure of the defect alone will often halt the progress of the aortic regurgitation.

5 Increased pulmonary vascular resistance occurs secondary to a high pulmonary blood flow at a high pressure. Heart failure is controlled but weight gain is poor. The hole remains large and there is apparent improvement over the next 12 months because the left-to-right shunt diminishes due to the increased resistance to blood flowing through the lungs.

It is important not to be misled by the apparent improvement in such cases, because if the defect is not closed before the age of 2 years changes in the lung vessels are unlikely to regress after surgery. Without surgery, pulmonary vascular disease develops, the shunt reverses, the patient becomes cyanosed and breathless and will die in the second or third decade. The only management of pulmonary vascular disease is prevention.

6 There is a small group of cases in which the defect is large but for some reason the pulmonary vascular resistance does not fall at birth, as it should. There is little or no shunting through the defect, there are few or no symptoms, and the pulmonary vascular resistance continues to rise and eventually pulmonary vascular disease results. Such patients are often not referred to cardiology units because they are relatively well as children.

Signs. The turbulence of blood flowing from the left to the right ventricle causes a systolic thrill and pan-systolic murmur at the left sternal edge, maximal in the third and fourth left interspaces. In moderate and large defects a diastolic murmur is audible at the cardiac apex due to excessive blood flow through a normal mitral valve.

X-ray. This may be normal in very small defects but the larger the defect the greater the degree of pulmonary plethora and the larger the heart. There is left ventricular enlargement and the pulmonary artery is prominent.

ECG. This shows biventricular hypertrophy.

Treatment. Medical treatment is used to control the heart failure and the defect is closed surgically using cardiopulmonary bypass if:

1 The infant fails to thrive despite medical treatment.

2 There is a danger of pulmonary vascular disease developing.

3 The patient has symptoms of excessive breathlessness and recurrent chest infections that interfere with schooling.

The majority of patients with small and moderate VSDs do not require surgery and most will close at some time even in adult life.

Patent ductus arteriosus

The natural history is related to the size of the ductus and to the changes that occur in the pulmonary circulation after birth. If the ductus does not close during the first 2 weeks of life in the full-term infant, spontaneous closure thereafter is rare.

Patients with a *small* ductus arteriosus have no symptoms and the only risk is of bacterial endarteritis. Before ducts were closed, the incidence of endarteritis was of the order of 9%. If the ductus is *large*, heart failure occurs in infancy. Referral of patients with large ducts is so common now that they are usually closed in infancy. If they are not closed and the patient survives, pulmonary vascular disease develops in the same way as in large ventricular septal defect. Similarly, there is a rare group of patients who have a large ductus but in whom the pulmonary vascular resistance remains high from birth and they never develop heart failure. They are often not referred until the shunt is reversed and they have cyanosis and clubbing of the toes and fingers of the left hand.

In premature infants, however, spontaneous closure may occur up to 3 months after birth, and often this is at the time that the child reaches maturity outside the uterus. Now that very premature babies survive by using ventilation, we are seeing another group of patients who develop heart failure secondary to a large shunt through the ductus, and it may be impossible to control the heart failure sufficiently to wean the child off the ventilator; such patients need to have the duct closed either by the use of indomethacin or surgically.

Signs. The pulses are collapsing due to the sudden leak of blood from the aorta to the pulmonary artery. If the ductus is large, the diastolic pressures in the aorta and pulmonary artery are equal and shunting occurs only during systole, and there is a systolic murmur only. In moderate- and small-sized ducts there is a pressure gradient between the aorta and pulmonary artery in systole and diastole, so the murmur is continuous. It has a machinery-like quality best heard in the pulmonary area and may be accompanied by a thrill. In moderate and large ducts an independent diastolic murmur is heard at the cardiac apex due to excessive flow through the mitral valve.

X-ray. This shows left ventricular enlargement, prominent pulmonary artery and pulmonary plethora.

ECG. This shows increase in left ventricular activity and there may be some increased right activity also if the duct is large.

Treatment. Heart failure if present is treated medically and the ductus closed surgically whenever it is diagnosed; the risk of surgery is very small and no greater in babies than in older children.

Atrial septal defect

It is uncommon for an atrial septal defect alone to cause symptoms in infancy. The resistance to filling in the two ventricles is the same and no blood flows through the defect. As the compliance of the right ventricle falls towards the end of the first year of life, left-to-right shunting begins. Only in large shunts are symptoms present in childhood: in the majority a heart murmur is discovered during routine examination and the patient has few or no symptoms. Symptoms occur in the second and third decades, pulmonary hypertension develops secondary to the large blood flow into the lungs, and heart failure and atrial arrhythmias result. As the pulmonary hypertension increases, the right ventricle hypertrophies and becomes less compliant and the flow through the defect reverses causing cyanosis. Infective endocarditis does not occur in simple secundum atrial septal defects.

Signs. There is heaving of the right ventricle due to increased blood volume and an ejection systolic murmur is heard in the pulmonary area due to excessive blood flow through a normal pulmonary valve. The second heart sound is widely split because it takes longer for the volume overloaded right ventricle to empty and the pulmonary valve closure is delayed. The wide splitting does not vary with respiration and is described as 'fixed'. In large defects, a diastolic murmur is audible in the tricuspid area due to excessive flow through the tricuspid valve.

X-ray. This shows pulmonary plethora, a prominent pulmonary artery and right ventricular enlargement: the apex of the heart is lifted up from the diaphragm.

ECG. This shows right ventricular hypertrophy with an rsR pattern in the right ventricular leads.

Treatment. Atrial septal defects should be closed surgically by school age. Cardiopulmonary bypass is necessary.

STENOTIC LESIONS

Coarctation of aorta
This condition presents at different ages depending on its severity.

1 Severe coarctation
When coarctation of the aorta is *severe*, acute symptoms occur in the neonatal period, most commonly during the second week of life. Many have associated cardiac lesions such as ventricular septal defect, aortic stenosis and mitral valve abnormalities. The site of the obstruction is usually above the ductus arteriosus, and as long as the duct remains patent blood will flow through it from the pulmonary artery to the lower half of the body: the fetal circulation is therefore maintained. When the duct closes, the left ventricle cannot maintain the flow of blood to the aorta below the site of the coarctation, and left ventricular failure results followed by right ventricular failure and renal failure. Unless treatment is given urgently, the child dies.

Signs. The baby is breathless, grey and collapsed with crepitations at lung bases and liver enlargement. The pulses are better in the arms than the legs but may be difficult to feel everywhere: the blood pressure is lower in the legs than the arms. The urinary output is poor and there may be anuria. There are no murmurs or a very soft systolic one in the pulmonary area.

X-ray. This shows generalized cardiac enlargement and congested lung fields.
ECG. This shows *right* ventricular hypertrophy.

The use of prostaglandins in these babies to re-open the ductus has improved their prognosis greatly. Renal flow is improved, diuretics are effective and heart failure can be controlled prior to urgent surgery. The ductus is ligated and the coarctation resected, using the subclavian flap technique which prevents re-coarctation in many cases.

2   Mild coarctation

These patients survive infancy without symptoms and gradually a collateral circulation develops; hypertension occurs in the head and arms. Of these patients, 50% would die by the age of 32 years if no treatment was given, and 75% by the age of 46 years.

Signs. The pulses in the arms and neck are normal, but the leg pulses are delayed and weak or absent. The blood pressure is raised in the arms and lower in the legs where the pulse pressure is reduced. Collateral vessels are rarely obvious clinically before the age of 6 years. They can be seen and felt down the medial borders of the scapulae and blowing systolic murmurs are heard over them.

X-ray. This shows left ventricular enlargement and in an overpenetrated film the aorta is seen bulging above the coarctation and there is post-stenotic dilatation below, giving a figure 3 shape.

ECG. This shows left ventricular dominance.

Treatment. Surgery is advised in all patients as soon as the diagnosis is made. The sooner the hypertension in the upper part of the body is relieved the better; there is evidence that the blood pressure will not return to normal if hypertension is allowed to persist too long. Balloon dilatation (p. 142) is used in suitable cases.

Aortic valve stenosis

The natural history varies with the severity of the narrowing. Children with a mild degree of stenosis have no symptoms and rarely deteriorate until adult life when calcification occurs on the valve and the stenosis becomes more severe. In mild stenosis with gradients of only 20 mmHg, no restrictions of exercise are necessary. It is becoming easier to monitor the gradients by Doppler echocardiography as the patients grow up. In critical stenosis however heart failure occurs in the first 2 weeks of life, and if the lesion is not recognized 50% die. In severe stenosis, syncope and dizziness are the first symptoms. The risk of sudden death is 1%. Infective endocarditis occurs in about 1% per annum and may be followed by progressive aortic regurgitation.

Signs. In children there are usually no thrills over the precordium but systolic thrills occurs in the suprasternal notch and over the right carotid artery. An ejection systolic murmur is best heard in the aortic area and conducted to the neck. In mild cases the pulses are normal, but in severe cases the pulses are of small volume.

X-ray. This shows a heart of left ventricular shape with normal vascularity of the lungs.

ECG. This shows left ventricular dominance and in severe cases there is T-wave inversion over the left ventricular leads.

Treatment. Surgery is advised when the gradient between the left ventricle and the aorta is more than 60 mmHg at rest. In childhood surgery is palliative only. The stenosis cannot be completely relieved or too much incompetence will result after cutting the valve. Parents must be warned that further surgery will be necessary in the future and eventually valve replacement is likely. Valvuloplasty (see below) is being used in suitable cases, but there is a risk of causing significant aortic regurgitation.

Pulmonary valve stenosis

The natural history varies with the severity of the stenosis. A mild stenosis is compatible with normal activities and a normal life expectation, and is unlikely to increase significantly during the patient's lifetime. In moderate stenosis, however, although there may be no symptoms, the stenosis becomes relatively greater as the patient grows and progressive hypertrophy of the right ventricular muscle occurs.

Severe stenosis is often well tolerated during childhood but eventually there is a limitation of cardiac output, and breathlessness, arrhythmias and heart failure occur. Critical pulmonary stenosis in infancy will cause early death unless recognized. Such infants usually have a right-to-left shunt at atrial level secondary to the severe hypertension in the right ventricle, and present with cyanosis and heart failure.

Signs. A systolic thrill and ejection systolic murmur occur in the second left interspace and the murmur is conducted to the left lung apex. There is heaving of the right ventricle because of the increased pressure and the pulmonary valve closure is delayed and soft, causing wide splitting of the second sound.

X-ray. This shows a prominent pulmonary artery (due to post-stenotic dilatation) and normal or reduced pulmonary vasculature peripherally.

ECG. This shows right ventricular hypertrophy and in severe cases also right atrial hypertrophy.

Treatment. The stenosis should be relieved when the pressure gradient between the right ventricle and pulmonary artery is greater than 60 mmHg at rest. This used to be done by open heart surgery but valvuloplasty is now the treatment of choice in isolated pulmonary valve stenosis.

Valvuloplasty and balloon dilatation

Catheters with balloons at their tips have been used for tearing the atrial septum in transposition of the great arteries, since 1966. Now there is a different type of balloon catheter which has a large diameter balloon which withstands high pressures. It can be used to dilate stenotic valves (valvuloplasty) and to relieve moderate stenosis in blood vessels. Valvuloplasty is now the treatment of choice for isolated pulmonary valve stenosis, but in aortic stenosis and coarctation of the aorta there is a higher risk of complications.

CYANOTIC LESIONS

Tetralogy of Fallot

After the first year of life this is the commonest cyanotic lesion. The natural history was not documented before surgical help became possible and will never now be accurately known. The outlook is related to the severity of the narrowing of the right ventricular outflow tract; the greater the narrowing the greater the right-to-left shunt and degree of cyanosis. Such patients are at risk from thrombosis, infective endocarditis, embolus and cerebral abscess. The lesion presents in two ways:

1 The onset of 'cyanotic attacks'. These occur suddenly without warning usually after 5 months of age. The child is well when he wakes up in the morning, has a normal breakfast then cries and screams in pain, becomes breathless and cyanosed, then rolls up his eyes and loses consciousness fleetingly. Although attacks may occur at other times of the day, the commonest is in the morning. Some of the most severe attacks occur in children who are virtually pink at rest.

2 Gradual increase in cyanosis at rest and on exertion. Squatting occurs on exertion and is diagnostic of tetralogy of Fallot.

Signs. The degree of cyanosis is variable but always increases dramatically on exertion. Clubbing of the fingers and toes should be looked for. Some children who are not obviously cyanosed at rest do have clubbing if they are active and are cyanosed the greater part of the day. There is increased heaving of the right ventricle and the systolic murmur is best heard in the second and third left interspaces. It is ejection in type and due to blood flowing through the narrowed infundibulum and pulmonary valve. Cardiac failure does not occur.

X-ray. This shows a heart of right ventricular shape with a hollow pulmonary bay and reduced vascularity of the lungs.

ECG. This shows right ventricular hypertrophy and right atrial hypertrophy.

Treatment. Cyanotic attacks are treated with oxygen and intravenous propranolol. They can be prevented by oral propranolol until surgery is performed.

A shunt operation is done in babies, usually a Blalock anastomosis between the subclavian artery and the pulmonary artery. Gore-Tex can be used to increase the size of the shunt. After the age of 1 year total correction is recommended unless the pulmonary arteries are small or deformed.

Transposition of the great arteries

This presents with cyanosis on the first day of life and the cyanosis increases as the ductus arteriosus closes: there are no murmurs. The child becomes breathless and unable to feed.

X-ray. This shows a heart with a narrow pedicle due to the aorta lying in front of the pulmonary artery. The shape of the heart is like an egg with the pointed part of the egg forming the apex of the heart. The lung fields are well vascularized.

ECG. This shows right ventricular hypertrophy.

Unless urgent treatment is given, these children die. The baby must be transferred to a special unit and balloon septostomy performed—a catheter with the deflated balloon is passed into the inferior vena cava from the femoral vein and advanced to the right atrium and through the foramen ovale to the left atrium. The balloon is then inflated with dye and pulled back sharply into the right atrium to tear the atrial septum. This allows mixing between the two sides of the heart. If necessary, prostaglandins can be used to open the ductus and increase the pulmonary blood flow, which results in an increased volume of blood returning to the left atrium and increases the shunt through the torn septum. The satisfactory tear can be seen on echocardiography.

Some time between 6 months and a year, surgery is carried out to redirect the systolic and pulmonary venous return so that oxygenated blood flows to the right ventricle and aorta, and deoxygenated blood to the left ventricle and the lungs. A relatively new operation is used in a few centres now in which the aorta and pulmonary artery are 'switched' so that they then arise from the correct ventricle.

CARDIAC FAILURE

Heart failure is a medical emergency. It occurs more commonly in the first 3 months of life than in any other period of childhood. The earlier in life it occurs, the worse the prognosis because it means the heart lesion is a severe one. It is usually due to congenital heart disease and is often precipitated by a chest infection. It is also caused by myocarditis and endocarditis.

The child is restless, fretful and looks anxious. There is tachypnoea, dyspnoea, tachycardia and sweating. The heart is enlarged and the liver is enlarged and tender. Crepitations occur at the lung bases. Oedema of the limbs comes later. In left ventricular failure there is a dry irritating cough. A gain of weight in a child who is not feeding well suggests fluid retention due to heart failure.

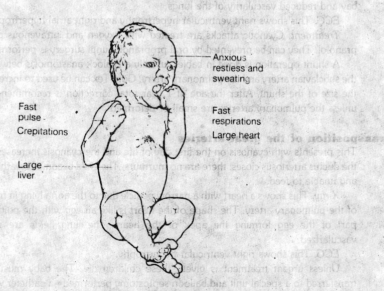

Anxious restless and sweating

Fast pulse
Crepitations

Fast respirations
Large heart

Large liver

Fig. 11.2. Cardiac failure in infancy.

Prompt treatment is essential:

1   Prop the child up as comfortably as possible and give oxygen in a concentration of 30%.

2   Sedate with phenobarbitone if the child is restless.

3   Correct any acidosis, hypoglycaemia, hypocalcaemia or anaemia.

4   Treat respiratory infection with antibiotics.

5   Nurse in a cool environment if there is a large left-to-right shunt (such children have a high metabolic rate).

6   Feed by oesophageal tube, starting with clear fluids.

7   Medication. Digoxin used to be used to increase the pumping action of the heart but has now been replaced by vasodilator drugs. These lower the systemic resistance and remove the load from the left ventricle. Captopril is the drug of choice.

Diuretics play an important part in therapy. Frusemide is safe and can be given orally, intravenously or intramuscularly. It is often combined with spironolactone to prevent potassium loss but if there is poor renal function, hyperkalaemia may occur.

Surgical treatment of congenital heart disease

As cardiac surgery advances there is a tendency to operate on the common lesions earlier in life. This often means operating before the child has any symptoms, but surgery is generally safer before the myocardium is damaged as a result of the defect and it is much more likely to return to normal after successful surgery as the child grows, so that in the long term myocardial function is normal.

Informing parents about heart disease

Parents are in a state of shock when they first hear that their child has heart disease. It is valuable therefore to provide them with some written information and a diagram of the particular problem in their child. They must be assured that it is no fault of theirs that the abnormality has occurred, and told that it took place in the first 6-10 weeks of pregnancy. They should be told that congenital heart disease is quite different from coronary artery disease and hypertension.

It is not necessary to restrict exercise in patients with congenital heart disease—the patients usually restrict themselves. The exception is in aortic stenosis and the problem is becoming easier now that gradients can be measured by echocardiography. If there are gradients of only 20 mmHg, restriction is not necessary, but if the gradient is higher yet not requiring surgery, competitive sports and cross-country running should be avoided.

Parents should be told of the danger of endocarditis and the necessity for prophylaxis with amoxycillin when dental treatment is required. Small defects where there is a jet effect through the hole and severely stenosed valves are more likely to be associated with endocarditis than are large defects and mildly stenosed valves.

ARRHYTHMIAS

The commonest arrhythmia in childhood is *supraventricular tachycardia*. It may rarely occur *in utero* and can be confirmed by fetal echocardiography, and controlled by treating the mother. Babies may be born in heart failure or develop heart failure as a result of such tachycardia. If it is not recognized the infants become acutely ill, collapsed and grey and need urgent help—in such cases the quickest treatment is to give a direct current shock. This can be performed under sedation or anaesthesia. If the child's condition is fairly good, propranolol should be given. It may produce hypotension and the blood pressure and electrocardiogram must be monitored. Prolonged treatment may be necessary to suppress attacks if they are frequent and prolonged.

Ventricular extrasystoles in childhood are not uncommon and, if an electrocardiogram shows these to be single, unifocal and abolished by exercise, they are not of serious significance. If however they occur in runs and are multifocal, further investigation and treatment are required.

Congenital heart block rarely requires treatment but if the heart rate is below 40/minute, if there are ventricular ectopic beats and heart failure, a pacemaker is necessary.

Episodes of *bradycardia and sinus arrest* are of serious import, particularly if there are episodes of loss of consciousness. Electrophysiological studies should be performed and a pacemaker inserted if necessary.

Rhythm problems are best investigated by ambulatory 24-hour ECG monitoring. It is used to confirm the diagnosis when necessary and to study the effect of treatment.

HYPERTENSION

Hypertension is less common in children than in adults: that fact together with the difficulty of its measurement (p. 38) causes it to remain undetected all too often. Blood pressure increases up to the age of 15 when adult levels are reached.

In general those children who have a blood pressure about the 90th centile in early life tend to remain at that end of the distribution curve in later childhood and probably adult life also. The blood pressure of any child has a close correlation with that of the parents and siblings. In childhood, there is no sex difference in blood pressure levels.

The important causes are of renal, adrenal (e.g. adrenogenital syndrome and Cushing's syndrome) or vascular (coarctation of the aorta) origin. Renal artery stenosis is exceedingly rare, but renal parenchymal diseases resulting from glomerulonephritis, pyelonephritis, or congenital defect, are relatively common, and are the chief contributors to severe hypertension, hypertensive encephalopathy and retinopathy.

Compared with adults who have hypertension, a primary cause is found much more often, and is itself more often totally correctable. For instance, unilateral kidney disease or coarctation if treated surgically early in life may abolish hypertension. However, 10–15% of children with hypertension do not yield a primary cause, and are then considered to have 'essential hypertension'.

Hypertension may be asymptomatic, or may present in a wide variety of ways—failure to thrive, fits, heart failure or, in the older child, headaches and malaise. Salt restriction, diuretics and hypotensive drugs are used as for adults—and tolerated rather better by most children.

FURTHER READING

Anderson RH. Macartney FJ. Shinebourne EA and Tynan M. *Paediatric Cardiology*. Churchill Livingstone.
Jordan SC and Scott O. *Heart Disease in Paediatrics*. Butterworth.

Chapter 12
The Respiratory Tract

Respiratory infections and allergy are important causes of morbidity and are common reasons for a child being taken to a doctor or admitted to hospital.

Certain problems are more common at certain ages as shown in Fig. 12.1. The same organism may cause different illnesses at different ages. For example, respiratory syncytial virus, which commonly causes lower respiratory tract illness (bronchiolitis) in infants, is more likely to cause a cold or a sore throat in older children.

Symptoms of respiratory tract disease

Cough in children usually has its origin in the upper respiratory tract (infection, allergy), less often in the lungs. It is usually easy to distinguish a 'throaty' from a 'chesty' cough: a barking cough suggests laryngeal or tracheal disease. Young asthmatics may cough instead of wheeze, especially at night. Children usually swallow their sputum unless it is copious. (Wheezing is discussed on p. 155, stridor on p. 151)

Earache is common with any upper respiratory catarrh as well as in otitis media. Pain from lower back teeth may be referred to the ear.

Epistaxis (nose bleed) usually originates from the anterior inferior corner of the nasal septum (Little's area). The commonest causes are minor injury and upper respiratory tract infections. The child may alarm everyone by vomiting blood which has been swallowed. Epistaxis may be a prodromal symptom of measles or rubella. First aid consists of sitting the child up and squeezing the nose firmly whilst the child is comforted and told to breathe through the mouth.

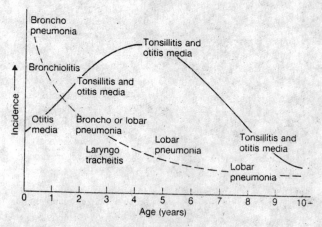

Fig. 12.1. The incidence of respiratory infections at different ages.

148

UPPER RESPIRATORY TRACT

Most illnesses of childhood are infections: most childhood infections are respiratory and involve only the upper respiratory tract. A wide variety of micro-organisms is involved, but the great majority are viral. The terms tonsillitis and otitis media are used if there is clear evidence of inflammation of the tonsils or middle ears, respectively. In the absence of tonsils (atrophied or removed), an inflamed throat is called pharyngitis.

The term 'upper respiratory tract infection' (URTI) is conventionally used to describe the equivalent of the common cold in young children. It presents with cough, anorexia and fever. In addition to nasal obstruction, the throat may be congested. Eustachian tube obstruction often causes earache and the eardrums may appear congested. Antibiotics are not indicated, but decongestant nose drops (e.g. 1/4% ephedrine in saline) before feeds will make it easier for babies to suck: paracetamol will reduce fever; both will relieve earache.

Infections of the upper respiratory tract are the usual precipitants of febrile convulsions (p. 106) and are sometimes the precursors of acute specific fevers, especially measles (p. 232).

Recurrent coughs and colds

Recurrent coughs and colds, sometimes with sore throat and earache, are very common in young children. Some babies and toddlers are catarrhal much of the time. If their colds spread to other members of the household and are worse in winter, they are probably viral. If they are non-seasonal and do not spread, they are probably of allergic origin. The first winter at school or nursery is frequently punctuated by upper respiratory infections.

Poor social circumstances predispose to catarrh. Some children will not blow their noses; some with severe nasal obstruction cannot. Cough persisting after pertussis may be due to lobar or segmental collapse. Night cough may be caused by a post-nasal drip (as with chronic sinus infection) or by mite sensitivity. Rarer causes of recurrent cough include cystic fibrosis, hiatus hernia and tuberculosis.

If the cause cannot be eliminated, decongestants and cough suppressants will give symptomatic relief. The best healer is the passage of time.

Otitis media

Acute otitis media is common throughout the first 8 years of childhood, and is generally associated with an infection of the nasopharynx. In the older child the cardinal symptom of earache makes detection easy. In infants it may not be so obvious. They usually have a high fever and are irritable, rolling their heads from side to side, or rubbing their ears.

At onset there may be just mild inflammation of the pars flaccida (the superior part of the tympanic membrane) with dilated vessels running down the handle of the malleus, and an absent light reflex. This progresses to a red bulging tympanic membrane which may perforate and discharge pus. This should be differentiated from the mildly pink dull drum that may be present in any child with an URTI.

In at least half the affected children, the cause will be viral. In the rest, the pathogens more frequently incriminated are *Streptococcus pneumoniae* and

Haemophilus influenzae. Ampicillin or amoxycillin are the antibiotics of choice, and paracetamol is invaluable for the fever and pain.

Mastoiditis, lateral sinus thrombosis, meningitis, and cerebral abscess are rare complications. Persistent aural discharge (chronic suppurative otitis media) is more common.

Secretory otitis media (glue ear, serous otitis media)

The accumulation of sticky serous material in the middle ear may arise insidiously or following acute otitis media. The symptoms are earache, deafness or a feeling of fullness or 'popping' in the ear. It is especially common in children who have atopy, frequent upper respiratory infections or cleft palate. The eardrum is usually dull and retracted. The malleus handle is more horizontal than usual and appears shorter, broader and whiter. The light reflex may be absent and a fluid level may be seen. There is usually conductive hearing loss. It occurs mainly below the age of 10 years when it is the commonest reason for hearing loss. Antibiotics, antihistamines and decongestant nose drops may be tried, but if there is significant deafness an indwelling tube (grommet) is inserted through the eardrum to aerate the middle ear and is left in for 6–12 months.

Any child who has otitis media must be followed up until the eardrum and hearing are normal. If response to treatment is slow or infections recur, an ear, nose and throat specialist should be consulted.

Tonsils and adenoids

Lymphoid tissue grows rapidly in the first 5 years of life. Tonsils and adenoids are usually small in infants and reach their greatest relative size between 4 and 7 years. Cervical glands are normally palpable at this age, and readily enlarge in response to local infection.

Acute tonsillitis

This is very common in the age group 2–8 years. It is uncommon in infants. There is sudden onset of fever, sore throat and dysphagia. Vomiting and abdominal pains are common in toddlers. The tonsils are enlarged and fiery red; exudate may appear later. The commonest pathogen to be cultured is beta-haemolytic streptococcus, but no bacterial pathogen can be identified in over half the cases. The presence of small petechiae on the palate or ulcers on the buccal mucosa or gums makes a viral aetiology more likely. Paracetamol and cool drinks provide symptomatic relief. Penicillin is often used because it will eradicate streptococci and reduce the risk of complications.

Complications are rare, but important; they may be immediate or delayed:
1 Immediate complications are as follows:
   (a) *Peritonsillar abscess* (quinsy) which is characterized by severe symptoms of tonsillitis and marked dysphagia. The tonsil appears displaced towards the midline with the anterior pillar of the fauces pushed forward.
   (b) *Cervical abscess.* Marked cervical adenitis is usual at the time of tonsillitis, but occasionally infection localizes in one of the cervical lymph glands to form an abscess. Early antibiotic treatment of peritonsillar or cervical abscess may produce cure, but once they are fully developed surgical drainage is required.

2   Delayed complications after certain streptococcal infections of the tonsil are as follows.
   (a) *Acute nephritis* (p. 195) 2–3 weeks after the infection.
   (b) *Rheumatic fever* (p. 182) 1–2 weeks after the infection (now very rare in developed countries).

Tonsillectomy

This operation is reserved chiefly for children over the age of 4 who have had recurrent bouts of acute tonsillitis (more than three a year), or persistent or chronic infection of the tonsils.

Parents seek the operation for a multiplicity of reasons. They need to be told that in general tonsillectomy does not prevent the child catching colds, sore throats or bronchitis; it does not improve the child's appetite or growth. Large healthy tonsils are only exceptionally big enough to obstruct swallowing or breathing.

Adenoidectomy

This is usually done at the same time as tonsillectomy. Indications for it to be done independently are recurrent otitis media, sinusitis or obstruction of the nasopharynx.

Sinusitis

The frontal and sphenoidal sinuses do not develop until 5 and 9 years, respectively. The maxillary and ethmoidal sinuses are small in these years and sinusitis is uncommon before the age of 5. Maxillary antra generally reflect nasal pathology (infection or allergy). Post-nasal drip may cause nocturnal or early morning cough.

Allergic rhinitis

The symptoms are recurrent bouts of sneezing with a watery nasal discharge and watering eyes which are worse when the child is outside in bright sunshine. The nose may be blocked, and inspection inside the nostril reveals pale oedematous mucosa. When it occurs in late spring and early summer in response to grass pollen, it is called *hay fever*, but it may occur in response to a variety of allergens including dust, animal dander and moulds. A careful history is more likely to identify the allergen than allergy tests. Avoidance of the allergen may not be possible. Sodium cromoglycate nose and eye drops are useful; a few children are helped by antihistamines.

Stridor

Stridor is noisy breathing originating from above the bronchi. It commonly originates from the larynx and is mainly inspiratory in timing.

The young child's larynx is not only relatively smaller, but the walls are flabby compared with the firm cartilaginous adult larynx. It is a voice bag not a voice box and it collapses and obstructs easily.

Congenital stridor

Stridor caused by abnormalities of the pharynx, larynx or trachea may be audible from birth. The least rare form. 'congenital laryngeal stridor'. is due to floppy aryepiglottic folds. It does not cause serious obstruction and gradually disappears as the laryngeal cartilage becomes firmer during the first year of life. If it is severe enough to cause intercostal and suprasternal recession. or if there is no improvement by the age of 3 months. laryngoscopy is advisable.

Acute stridor

Acquired stridor in children of 5 years or over is nearly always due to viral laryngitis and can be managed safely at home. In younger children, especially in infants and toddlers. stridor can progress to serious respiratory obstruction and thence to respiratory arrest with alarming rapidity. Hospital admission is therefore mandatory. The main causes of acute stridor are:

1 Acute laryngotracheitis.
2 Epiglottitis.
3 Foreign body in the larnyx.

Acute laryngotracheitis

This is common from 1 to 4 years. alarming and potentially dangerous. There is sudden onset. often at night. of stridor. harsh cry and a barking cough (croup). There is moderate fever and systemic illness. In addition to stridor there may be intercostal and suprasternal indrawing if obstruction is marked. The fauces may be mildly inflamed. A raised respiratory rate and abnormal signs in the lungs suggest that the lower respiratory tract is also involved. Laryngotracheitis is of viral origin so antibiotics are not needed. Cold humidity gives symptomatic relief. Sedation lessens anxiety and may help the breathing. In severe cases blood gases should be monitored. and ventilation may be necessary.

Epiglottitis

This also presents as acute stridor. but the child is acutely ill and feverish. He prefers to sit up: drooling is common because swallowing is difficult. The swollen epiglottis may be seen like a cherry when the pharynx is examined and may be seen on a soft-tissue lateral X-ray of the neck. but both procedures may precipitate respiratory arrest and should not be undertaken without facilities for resuscitation. The cause is infection with *Haemophilus influenzae* which may be cultured from blood. Prompt antibiotic and supportive treatment are essential.

Laryngeal foreign body

There is stridor of acute onset but the child is otherwise well. There may be a history of a choking episode. X-ray will reveal a radio-opaque object but laryngoscopy may be needed for diagnosis as well as for treatment.

Apnoea

Temporary cessation of breathing is a frightening occurrence. It can result from central respiratory depression or from mechanical obstruction (including the inhalation of food or vomit). It may occur during the first day or two of respiratory infections. particularly pertussis or respiratory syncytial virus. However. many infants are rushed to hospital by their parents, who believe their child has stopped breathing. Often it is not clear whether anxious parents have merely misinterpreted the normal variable breathing of a small baby, or whether the baby genuinely has had a significant spell of apnoea. When the apnoea is associated with cyanosis, or unconsciousness. the differential diagnosis must include a seizure or congenital heart disease. For very worried parents the loan of an apnoea alarm. which sounds when the baby stops breathing, may be comforting. There is no evidence that apnoea alarms lessen the incidence of sudden infant death syndrome (p. 246). Most children who die suddenly and unexpectedly in early life have not had previous spells of apnoea.

Influenza

Influenza tends to occur in epidemics. affecting particularly school children and young adults. The general symptoms of high fever. headache and malaise tend to overshadow the dry cough and sore throat. though there may be signs of pharyngitis, tracheitis or bronchitis. The main complications result from secondary bacterial infection of lungs. middle ear or sinuses.

The brief incubation period and high infectivity favour massive outbreaks in institutions such as boarding schools. The large number of strains. as well as the frequency of mutation involving the three types of myxovirus influenzae. make immunization of limited value. Treatment is symptomatic.

LOWER RESPIRATORY TRACT

The bronchial tree and its blood supply are present by the 20th week of gestation. and thereafter only enlarge. In contrast. the alveoli increase in number from 20 million at birth to the adult complement of 300 million. Respiratory disease in early childhood may therefore interfere with future lung development as well as causing direct lung damage.

The airways of an infant are particularly liable to obstruction. A tiny amount of mucus or a small degree of bronchospasm may narrow the airway dangerously. leading to poor oxygenation or collapse of a lung segment.

Bronchitis and bronchiolitis

Acute bronchitis occurs at all ages and is characterized by cough. fever and often wheezing. It is a common early feature of measles and whooping cough. Chronic bronchitis does not occur in children.

Bronchiolitis is confined to infants: the peak age is 4 months. Most cases are caused by respiratory syncytial virus and occur in winter epidemics. Older members of the household merely have mild upper respiratory tract symptoms. Bronchiolitis develops suddenly: in the morning the infant may be just a bit snuffly, but by afternoon he is irritable. coughing and breathless. The respiratory rate is high and. as respiratory distress increases. cyanosis may appear. Widespread high pitched rhonchi and crepitations can be heard throughout the lungs. The infant should be admitted to hospital where skilled nursing. oxygen and artificial ventilation are available. Antibiotics are often given as it is difficult to distinguish from pneumonia. Nasogastric tube feeding is likely to be needed for the very breathless infant, and careful attention has to be paid to fluid and calorie intake. After 2-3 days recovery gradually occurs. Up to half the infants diagnosed as having bronchiolitis subsequently develop recurrent wheezing (asthma).

Pneumonia

Bronchopneumonia

This is commonest in young children (Fig. 12.1) and in older children with some chronic condition affecting respiratory function (cystic fibrosis, congenital heart disease, severe cerebral palsy). A wide variety of organisms can be responsible: in the infant respiratory syncytial virus is the most important. It commonly follows bronchitis, measles and whooping cough. The onset is acute with rapid breathing, dry cough, fever and fretfulness. Generalized crepitations and rhonchi are usually present. Cyanosis occurs in severe cases and infants may develop cardiac failure. Chest X-ray often shows small patches of consolidation.

Hospitalization is usually needed. Oxygen and a broad-spectrum antibiotic are given. Gentle physiotherapy helps to moblilize secretions. Infants may need tube feeding initially.

Lobar pneumonia

This afflicts the 4-10-year-old child, and presents with sudden illness and high fever. Pleuritic pain may be felt in the chest, causing the child to lean towards the affected side, or may be referred to the abdomen or neck. The child is sick, looks flushed, breathes fast with an expiratory grunt and is using the alae nasi. There may be a 'cold sore' (Herpes simplex) on the lip. The respiratory rhythm may be reversed so that the pause comes after inspiration rather than expiration. There may be no cough. The clinical signs of consolidation may not be present at first but repeated examination will usually reveal them. A transient pleural rub is common. Lobar consolidation, with or without pleural effusion, is usually evident on X-ray.

Lobar pneumonia is usually caused by Strep. pneumoniae and penicillin achieves dramatic improvement within 24 hours. Provided that conditions are reasonable, this is a safe and rewarding condition to treat at home. It is best to give the initial dose of penicillin by injection as an ill child is likely to vomit medicine. A hypnotic will ensure sleep for the child and, if there is a troublesome cough, a cough-suppressant is given. Fluid intake is more important than food. Paracetamol and tepid sponging help reduce fever.

If signs or symptoms are still present after a week, careful examination including chest X-ray should be repeated to exclude such complications as pleural effusion or lobar collapse.

Staphylococcal pneumonia

This is a severe form of pneumonia which affects infants and children with cystic fibrosis. It is characterized by lung cysts on X-ray, and the sudden appearance of empyema or pneumothorax clinically. Lobar consolidation in an infant may be the first radiological sign. Prolonged treatment is required with an antibiotic effective against penicillin-resistant staphylococci.

Inhaled foreign bodies

Babies and toddlers are most at risk, for they tend to put everything into their mouths. Older children sometimes accidentally inhale objects during games or whilst stuffing their mouths too full of peanuts or sweets.

A foreign body may lodge at any level. At the time the child will cough, splutter or make choking noises but the episode is quickly forgotten and may not come out in the history without specific questioning. In the larynx an object is likely to cause a croupy cough and stridor (p. 151). If it passes through the larynx, it will lodge in a bronchus (right middle lobe or a lower lobe most often) and there will be no symptoms for a few days until infection, collapse or (less often) obstructive emphysema develop.

Whenever the possibility of a foreign body is suspected, both anteroposterior and lateral X-rays of the neck and chest should be taken. Translucent objects may not show and the search may have to be continued by direct laryngoscopy and bronchoscopy, which would in any case be required to remove the object.

THE WHEEZY CHILD

Wheezing is an obstructive respiratory sound arising in the smaller branches of the bronchial tree: on auscultation, rhonchi can be heard. They are most marked in expiration because the bronchial tree dilates in inspiration. The obstruction results from bronchospasm, mucosal oedema and secretions: babies wheeze readily because their airways are small. Bronchospasm results from the release of spasmogens (e.g. histamine, serotonin) from the bronchial mucosal cells. Mucosal oedema may be of allergic or infective origin. The appearance of the nasal mucosa often reflects what is happening lower down the respiratory tract.

Recurrent wheezing is common in childhood. Some young children outgrow this phase of 'wheezy bronchitis', but others continue to have recurrent bouts of wheezing and eventually are diagnosed as having asthma.

Asthma

This is characterized by recurrent bouts of wheezing, breathlessness and cough due to intermittent, reversible obstruction of the peripheral airways. It tends to occur in response to a variety of stimuli, and most often in children with a personal or family history of allergy.

It is important to try to understand the underlying factors in each wheezy child if the best help is to be given. The principal factors are as follows:

1 *Infection*. Bronchitis is common in young children and is often accompanied by wheezing (wheezy bronchitis). Wheezing is always a conspicuous feature of bronchiolitis. Infection is likely to be an important factor in those asthmatics who have most trouble in winter.

2 *Allergy*. Many asthmatics are sensitive to inhaled allergens, most commonly house dust mite or grass pollens. Allergens can be best identified from the history (e.g. wheezing at night or in the pollen season). A family history of allergies is common.

3 *Atopy*. The atopic state is defined as an altered body response to foreign proteins. IgE is produced readily in response to common environmental antigens. It has a strong genetic basis and commonly manifests as asthma, eczema and/or

hay fever. In the family history atopy and allergy often overlap.

4   Emotions. Exceptionally, a severe emotional upset may precipitate a first attack of wheezing. Commonly, excitement or anxiety can precipitate attacks in known asthmatics. Wheezing, especially if severe, causes anxiety and hence a bad attack may become self-perpetuating.

5   Exertion. Many asthmatics become wheezy on exertion, especially if it involves running. Exercise-induced wheezing occurs most readily in a cold atmosphere.

6   Atmosphere. Dusty air, 'stuffy' and smoke-filled rooms, or changes in air temperature may all precipitate wheezing.

In young children, upper respiratory tract infections appear to be the commonest precipitating factor, but as the child grows up others may become apparent—specific allergens, exercise, emotional upsets and changes of weather or environment.

Incidence

Up to 10% of infants have a tendency to wheeze in the first 2 years of life. Most grow out of it. About 3% of schoolchildren have asthma compared with 1% of adults, which suggests that many outgrow their asthma.

Clinical features

There is often a family history of asthma, eczema or hay fever; and the child may have had, or develop, other hypersensitivity phenomena. Eczema is particularly common from 1 to 8 years of age, and hay fever in the schoolchild.

In the early years, the child suffers from recurrent respiratory infections which persist longer than usual. Colds 'go to the chest', coughs persist, and the parents may notice wheezing. The wheezing may steadily worsen for a day or two before gradually improving. As the child becomes older, the bouts become more clearly defined and more strikingly intermittent. The onset is sudden, and the child starts wheezing or coughing; breathlessness increases and with it fear. On examination, the respiratory rate is increased and the child may be using the accessory muscles of respiration or pushing his hands against a table to force air out in expiration. The wheeze is mainly expiratory and on auscultation prolonged expiratory rhonchi are heard. Crepitations are variable.

Between attacks there are usually no symptoms or signs. Some children with frequent severe attacks develop hyperinflation and limited exercise tolerance. Useful indicators of severity are peak expiratory flow rate, days missed from school and weight gain.

Management

1   Prevention

The aim is to reduce the frequency and severity of attacks and to give the child and family confidence that they can cope with attacks without disruption of home or school life. Precipitating factors should always be sought (Fig. 12.2). In all cases it is worth reducing the child's exposure to common allergens such as

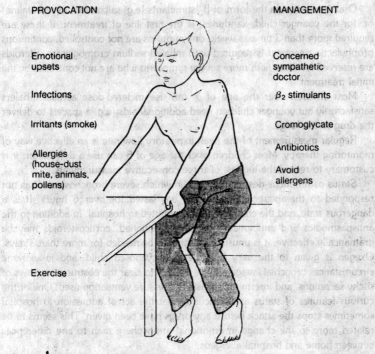

PROVOCATION	MANAGEMENT
Emotional upsets	Concerned sympathetic doctor
Infections	β_2 stimulants
Irritants (smoke)	Cromoglycate
	Antibiotics
Allergies (house-dust mite, animals, pollens)	Avoid allergens
Exercise	

Fig. 12.2. Precipitating factors in childhood asthma and possible solutions.

house-dust mite. The bedroom should be damp-dusted regularly, a plastic mattress cover used and pets banned from the bedroom.

Those at home are advised not to smoke in the house, particularly in the child's bedroom. Emotional problems at home or school can often be helped, but asthma generates its own emotional problems for the family. It can be a frightening condition for the child and family.

If asthmatic attacks are infrequent, medication is best reserved for symptomatic relief. If attacks are frequent and easily provoked, regular prophylaxis is helpful. Between these two, prophylaxis may be appropriate in specific circumstances e.g. before exercise.

2   Relief of wheezing

A mild attack will often respond to either inhaled or oral β_2-adrenoceptor stimulants. Clear instructions must be given and written down to limit the amount used.

Severe attacks must be stopped promptly. In hospital nebulized salbutamol is effective, and nebulizers can be issued for home use for children with severe asthma. Whenever asthma appears to have been precipitated by infection, antibiotics are often given, though viruses are usually responsible.

Oral medication in the form of β_2 stimulants (e.g. salbutamol or terbutaline) or, for the younger child, xanthines, is the first line of treatment. If these are required more than 3 times a week, or symptoms are not controlled, continuous prophylactic treatment is required with inhaled sodium cromoglycate. Steroids are reserved for those with more severe symptoms who are not controlled by the initial treatment.

Most children over the age of 7 can use metered-dose aerosol inhalers satisfactorily but younger children need additional aids (e.g. a spacer) to deliver the drug to the lungs.

Regular measurement of the peak expiratory flow rate is an effective way of monitoring therapy. Most children over the age of 5 can use a flow meter; it is customary to record the highest of three consecutive measurements.

Status asthmaticus describes a state in which severe bronchospasm has not responded to therapeutic measures, or has lasted for over 6 hours. It is a dangerous state, and the child should be admitted to hospital. In addition to the antispasmodics and antibiotics previously mentioned, corticosteroids may be dramatically effective; it is unusual for them to be needed for more than 3 days. Oxygen is given to the very breathless or cyanosed child, and in extreme circumstances bronchial lavage may be needed to clear the obstructed airways of sticky secretions, and intermittent positive pressure ventilation used. One of the curious features of status asthmaticus is that the act of admission to hospital sometimes stops the attack before any drugs have been given. This seems to be related more to the change in emotional atmosphere than to any differences between home and hospital allergens.

Asthma still causes a number of childhood deaths, usually when the attack has lasted several hours. Apart from mortality, the morbidity needs to be considered. Repeated attacks of asthma may lead to pulmonary complications, particularly hyperinflation and recurrent infection. Increasing kyphosis may further restrict respiration. Growth may be restricted and educational and social problems arise. Family life can be completely overshadowed by the fact that one child has asthma. This should be rare; asthma is a challenge that the doctor can help the family to overcome with the help of modern therapy.

FURTHER READING

Phelan PD Landau LI and Olinsky A. *Respiratory Illness in Children*. Blackwell Scientific Publications.

Chapter 13
The Alimentary Tract

Like most childhood illness, alimentary tract disorders are usually acute and infective. These are most serious in infancy, when fluid and electrolyte balance can become dangerously disturbed within a matter of hours and cause death or brain damage if not recognized and treated. Intestinal obstructions are also important and may be of congenital origin or acquired. Less common, but equally important, are malabsorption states including coeliac disease and cystic fibrosis. In children, peptic ulcers, ulcerative colitis and Crohn's disease are uncommon, and neoplasm very rare.

SYMPTOMS

The principal symptoms of acute alimentary disease are vomiting, diarrhoea and abdominal pain: of chronic disease, failure to thrive and diarrhoea. Constipation is a feature of acute intestinal obstruction, but chronic constipation and recurrent abdominal pain are not commonly due to structural alimentary tract disease. Abdominal distension is a feature of some acute and some chronic disorders.

Vomiting

It is very common for babies to bring up a small amount of food when breaking wind after a feed. This is *possetting*, a normal process that may be confused with vomiting by an inexperienced mother. Possetting is not accompanied by other symptoms, the baby is happy and gains weight well. Significant vomiting (Table 13.1) will be accompanied by weight loss, or at least an inadequate weight gain. Forceful (projectile) vomiting suggests high intestinal obstruction.

Haematemesis is not a common symptom. Small amounts of fresh or altered blood in the vomitus are seen if blood from the nose or throat has been swallowed, and with gastritis and oesophagitis. Massive haematemesis may also result from swallowed blood (e.g. after tonsillectomy), or from oesophageal or gastric varices or peptic ulcer. If the history raises the possibility of recent haematemesis but is not conclusive, check the stools for occult blood.

Diarrhoea and constipation

A history of diarrhoea or constipation should not be accepted without detailed enquiry. The number and consistency of stools passed by children, especially infants, is very variable and is influenced by diet. Breast-fed babies pass loose, bright yellow, odourless stools, usually 3 or 4 times a day and often after every feed but sometimes as infrequently as once as week. Bottle-fed babies pass paler, more acid stools which smell and may be quite hard, causing the baby to strain when defaecating. Unless this straining causes pain or rectal bleeding, or the bowels are being opened less than once a day, this should not be called

Table 13.1. Causes of vomiting.

Feeding errors:
1 In infants. too much food. too little food. the wrong kind of food.
   or faulty feeding technique
2 In older children. dietary indiscretions

Infections:
1 Gastritis (with or without enteritis)
2 Parenteral infections (e.g. tonsillitis. meningitis)
3 Acute appendicitis

Mechanical causes:
1 Intestinal obstruction. congenital or acquired
2 Hiatus hernia. oesophageal reflux

Raised intracranial pressure:
1 Meningitis. encephalitis
2 Space-occupying lesions (tumour. abscess. haematoma)

Metabolic disorders:
1 Intolerance of or allergy to food components (e.g. gluten. lactose.
   cow's milk protein)
2 Inborn errors of metabolism
3 Adrenal insufficiency
4 Ketosis. uraemia

Psychological problems:
1 Periodic syndrome ('cyclical vomiting'). migraine
2 Rumination

Miscellaneous:
1 Travel sickness
2 Poisoning

constipation. Many toddlers and some older children continue to have three or four bowel actions a day. after meals ('toddler diarrhoea'). If the stool consistency and weight gain are satisfactory. this is not abnormal. Frequent stools are often associated with a rapid transit time. and undigested food may be recognized in the stool within a few hours of being eaten (our personal best was carrots at 20 minutes). Chronic constipation (p. 129) may lead to faecal impaction and soiling. which may be mistakenly interpreted as diarrhoea. The principal causes of diarrhoea are shown in Table 13.2.

Abdominal pain

This is an important symptom but does not necessarily indicate abdominal disease. Acute central abdominal pain and vomiting are, for example. common symptoms of tonsillitis in young children. Recurrent abdominal pain may be a symptom of emotional stress. From about the age of 2 years. children can indicate the site of a pain. In infants. abdominal pain may be inferred from spasms of crying. restlessness and drawing up the knees. It is a very common symptom throughout childhood and is usually of no serious significance. The presence of

Table 13.2. Causes of diarrhoea.

Feeding errors:
1 In infants, too much food, too little or the wrong kind
2 In older children, dietary indiscretion

Inflammatory lesions:
1 Enteritis, including dysentery
2 Ulcerative colitis, Crohn's disease
3 Giardiasis (lambliasis)
4 Parenteral infections

Malabsorption states:
1 Steatorrhoea (coeliac disease, cystic fibrosis)
2 Disaccharide intolerance
3 Protein-losing enteropathy

Food intolerance

vomiting, bowel disturbance or fever in association with abdominal pain should prompt a more detailed appraisal, with re-examination after a few hours.

Abdominal distension

Abdominal distension can be difficult to assess because of the great normal variation. Fat babies appear to have bigger tummies than thin, muscular babies. Toddlers are normally rather pot-bellied in comparison with older children and black children in comparison with white. The mother will usually be able to say whether the abdomen is swollen.

Dehydration and wasting

It is important to recognize dehydration and wasting, especially in infants. Clinical dehydration results from inadequate fluid intake (which is not common) or excessive loss by vomiting, diarrhoea or polyuria. The combination of diarrhoea and vomiting, which is inevitably accompanied by inadequate intake, leads to losses of fluid and eletrolytes. This is seen in its most dramatic form in infantile gastroenteritis ('D and V'). The anterior fontanelle and the eyes become sunken, the skin loses its normal elasticity, the infant has an anxious look, a persistent cry and is restless. If the condition progresses, the baby becomes quiet and still, with sunken abdomen and signs of peripheral circulatory failure. In the older child, the lips and tongue become dry, and the eyes a little sunken. After infancy, vomiting rapidly leads to ketosis which is recognized by the smell of the breath and acidotic breathing, and the presence of ketones in the urine.

THE MOUTH

The teeth

The ages of usual appearance of the teeth are listed on p. 25. There is considerable normal variation in the time of eruption of teeth which may lead to unnecessary worry. The first teeth are sometimes apparent at birth, or no teeth may be cut until after the first birthday. Such extreme variations are usually physiological. Preventive dental health is important for all children, especially the handicapped. Caries are primarily microbial in origin, but dietary carbohydrate, particularly sucrose, is an important facilitator. Thus it is important to avoid frequent sugary food, especially in early life; medicines or vitamin drops containing sugar; and dummies soaked in sweet fluid. An adequate fluoride intake halves dental decay. In regions with low levels of fluoride in the water supply, toothpastes containing fluoride are recommended at least until the age of 16. For young children, fluoride drops or tablets are advised. Regular tooth-cleaning and dental supervision should be encouraged.

It is good practice for the doctor to include the teeth in the examination of the mouth. It gives an opportunity for either congratulation or health education, and occasionally an unexpected alveolar abscess is found to explain a persistent fever or ill health.

Cleft lip and palate

Although cleft lip is often called hare lip, the lesion is not usually central but may be unilateral or bilateral. It results from failure of fusion of the maxillary and frontonasal processes. In bilateral cases the premaxilla is anteverted (Fig. 13.1). There is always an associated nasal deformity. Early orthodontic treatment restores the normal anatomical relationships of the facial structures and simplifies surgical repair at about 3 months.

Cleft palate may occur alone or with cleft lip. It results from failure of fusion of the palatine processes and the nasal septum. Orthodontic treatment helps to align these structures and to stimulate palatal growth pending repair before the first birthday. Pending repair, special feeding techniques are often necessary. Submucous cleft palate, in which the muscle of the soft palate is cleft but the overlying mucosa is intact, is much less common. It may cause nasal regurgitation of feeds, and later 'cleft palate speech' because of nasal escape. The cleft can be seen as a dark line down the centre of the soft palate and the uvula is bifid. All varieties of cleft palate may be associated with deafness.

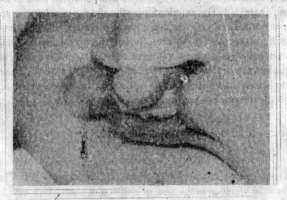

Fig. 13.1. Bilateral cleft lip

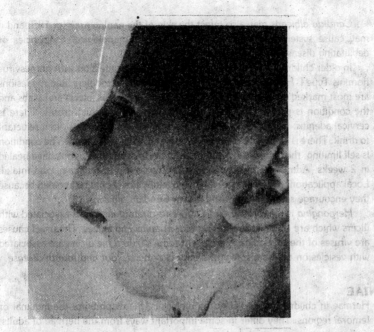

Fig. 13.2. An infant with micrognathia and retrognathia.

Micrognathia and retrognathia

Some babies are born with receding jaws. the jaw being either underdeveloped or displaced backward (Fig. 13.2). In severe cases. the tongue (which is also abnormally far back) obstructs breathing from birth. Most are self-correcting but the infant may need to be nursed prone in early life. Micrognathia may be associated with cleft palate. a combination which calls for very careful nursing. The term Pierre–Robin syndrome is often used to describe this combination. although the original papers do not mention cleft palate.

Stomatitis

In infancy. stomatitis is usually due to *Candida albicans* (monilia: thrush). This may develop in any baby whose feeds. bottles. teats or dummy have not been adequately sterilized. in babies who have been given broad-spectrum antibiotics. even for a few days only. and in emaciated and very ill infants. It appears as tiny white flecks inside the cheeks. on the tongue and on the roof of the mouth. The only possible source of diagnostic confusion is milk curds which are usually larger than thrush lesions. and can easily be detached with a spatula. *Candida albicans* will be cultured in large numbers from a swab (but it should be noted that this organism can often be cultured from the mouths or throats of healthy children). Treatment is aimed first at the cause (correction of faulty sterilization techniques or review of antibiotic policy) and second at elimination of the organism by the local application of nystatin It is important to continue local application for a few days after apparent cure. otherwise recurrence is likely.

Candida albicans may also infect the skin of the napkin area (p. 185) and it may cause systemic infection in children with immunological deficiencies or debilitating diseases.

In older children, stomatitis is usually due to a first infection with herpesvirus hominis Type I. *Herpetic stomatitis* is most common in toddlers, and the lesions are most marked on the lips and tongue. There are vesicles, ulcers and scabs and the condition is painful, the gums are inflamed and the child drools. There is cervical adenitis. Because of the pain the child will not eat and is often reluctant to drink. There is general misery, listlessness and a low-grade fever. The condition is self-limiting; the discomfort eases after a few days, and the lesions have healed in 2 weeks. Admission to hospital may be necessary to maintain fluid intake. Local applications are of limited value and antibiotics should be avoided because they encourage superadded infection with *Candida albicans*.

Herpangina is the term given to upper respiratory infections associated with ulcers which are confined to the posterior pharynx and fauces. The usual causes are viruses of the Coxsackie A group. In some children the ulcers are associated with vesicles on the hands, feet and buttocks—*hand, foot and mouth disease*.

HERNIAE

Herniae in children may involve the umbilicus, the diaphragm, the inguinal or femoral regions. They differ in some important ways from the herniae of adults.

Umbilical hernia

This is common and harmless. There is a small, sharply defined, circular defect in the centre of the umbilicus through which protrudes a small loop of bowel. Umbilical herniae are always easily reducible and virtually never strangulate. Spontaneous cure is usual before the first birthday though it may take up to 5 years. Treatment is not required. Babies with an umbilical hernia may cry (as may babies without hernia) but the hernia should not be regarded as the cause of the crying. In *para-umbilical hernia*, the orifice is usually immediately above the centre of the umbilicus. This may not heal spontaneously, and surgical repair will be required before the child starts school.

Diaphragmatic hernia

The most serious type of diaphragmatic hernia results from the failure of one or other leaf of the diaphragm (rarely both) to develop. It is more common on the left side and the lung on the side of the hernia is usually grossly underdeveloped. The hemithorax contains abdominal viscera, the heart is displaced to the opposite side, and the contralateral lung is compressed by the mediastinum. There is therefore grave respiratory difficulty from the moment of birth. If the hernia is left-sided, examination reveals the heart beat on the right side of the chest; if on the right, the apex beat is in the left axilla. Percussion note and air entry may be abnormal, but it is unusual to hear bowel sounds except with small herniae that gradually develop over a few days. A chest X-ray makes the diagnosis clear. Early intubation and positive pressure ventilation are usually necessary to maintain life until surgical repair can be undertaken.

Hiatus hernia associated with congenital short oesophagus is more common but less serious. The gastro-oesophageal junction is in the thorax, so that the anti-reflux effect of intra-abdominal pressure on the terminal oesophagus is lost. Thus there is both a partial thoracic stomach *and* gastro-oesophageal reflux. It presents with vomiting in early infancy, sometimes in the neonatal period; there may be a small amount of fresh or altered blood in the vomitus. The vomiting is not projectile, and weight gain is usually maintained. The diagnosis may be confirmed radiogically by giving a contrast meal. A small knuckle of stomach can be demonstrated above the diaphragm. In the head-down position, oesophageal reflux can be demonstrated; endoscopic evaluation of the degree of oesophagitis is desirable. Conservative management is indicated in the first instance, which consists of nursing the baby in the sitting position in a baby seat, thickening milk feeds and introducing solid foods as early as possible; antacids, domperidone or cimetidine are given. Remission of the symptoms can be anticipated towards the end of the first year of life. Exceptionally, a large hiatus hernia causes copious vomiting, weight loss or recurrent respiratory problems from inhalation, or is associated with persisting oesophagitis. Surgical correction is required.

Reflux (resulting from gastro-oesophageal incompetence) without a partial thoracic stomach is much more common and less serious. The messy possetting of milk after feeds in the early months of life is more of a nuisance than a threat to health; parental reassurance and thickened feeds are the only requirements. Resolution occurs by the age of 1 year.

Inguinal hernia

This is common in boys, rare in girls. It is often bilateral. A big hernia will form a large swelling in the scrotum, which can be reduced quite easily if the baby is quiet. A small hernia will cause a swelling in the groin which may be visible intermittently. The smaller the hernia, the more liable it is to strangulate. The doctor should therefore be more concerned about the hernia he cannot see than the one he can. In either case, the danger is present and spontaneous cure is not to be anticipated. Surgical repair should be undertaken at the first convenient moment.

INTESTINAL OBSTRUCTION

Intestinal obstruction may be present at birth, usually as a consequence of malformations of the alimentary tract, or may develop at any age thereafter. The cardinal symptoms are vomiting, abdominal distension, constipation, and (in children old enough to make their feelings clear) pain. Vomiting will lead to fluid and electrolyte loss with clinical signs of dehydration, and later to circulatory failure. Successful treatment therefore depends upon early diagnosis, adequate pre-operative correction of fluid and electrolyte loss, and skilled surgery and anaesthesia.

1 In the newborn

The level of the obstruction in the newborn may be anywhere from the oesophagus to the anus. Because swallowing by the fetus is one of the normal routes of disposal of amniotic fluid, obstruction may lead to accumulation of excess fluid (polyhydramnios) before birth, thus providing a diagnostic clue. The higher the level of obstruction, the more likely is this to occur. It is therefore common with oesophageal atresia but rare with rectal atresia. (Stenosis means narrowing of a passage; atresia means the passage has never been formed).

Oesophageal atresia is usually associated with tracheo-oesophageal fistula (Fig. 13.3) so that the bowel is soon filled with air via the fistula. In the absence of a fistula, the bowel remains airless and the abdomen sunken. Because swallowing is impossible, mucus tends to accumulate in the pharynx, and the infant after birth needs frequent aspiration of secretions. True vomiting is impossible, as food cannot reach the stomach, but if feeding is attempted, there will be immediate regurgitation and inhalation of feeds, with choking and cyanosis. Milk in the lungs causes severe pneumonia, and diagnosis should be made before feeding. If there has been polyhydramnios, or if suspicions are aroused by excess secretions, a nasogastric tube should be passed to demonstrate patency of the oesophagus. If this proves impossible, radiography after the careful instillation of a few millilitres of contrast medium into the oesophageal pouch will confirm the diagnosis and demonstrate the level of the obstruction. Early diagnosis and skilled surgery offer the best chance of cure, but there are other severe defects in about half the cases. Oesophageal and rectal atresia sometimes occur in the same baby.

Atresias at lower levels will cause vomiting and distension. If the obstruction is high, vomiting will be early. The vomit will contain bile because the obstruction is usually below the ampulla of Vater. Distension will be mainly epigastric. If the obstruction is lower, the vomiting will start a little later and the distension will be more generalized. *Duodenal atresia* and stenosis are particularly common in Down's syndrome. *Rectal atresia* is usually associated with fistula between the rectum and some part of the genito-urinary tract. An infant with low, complete obstruction cannot pass meconium, but small quantities may be passed by those with high obstruction.

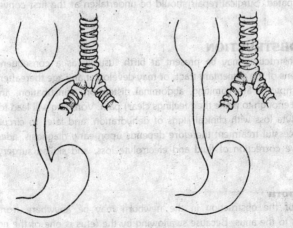

Fig. 13.3. Tracheo-oesophageal fistula before and after surgical correction.

In *Hirschsprung's disease*, obstruction is incomplete and is due to a narrow aganglionic segment of bowel, most commonly in the rectosigmoid region. Rectal biopsy yields the diagnosis. *Meconium ileus* is a manifestation of cystic fibrosis (p. 170). In *malrotation*, the bowel has become twisted at the time of reduction of the normal umbilical hernia of embryonic life and obstruction results from peritoneal bands.

There are many other causes of congenital obstruction, and often the precise anatomical diagnosis can only be made at operation. The site of obstruction may be deduced from the distribution of intestinal gas seen on a straight radiograph taken with the baby vertical.

In *exomphalos* (omphalocele) the temporary umbilical hernia of normal embryonic development has become permanent, and the baby is born with a variable amount of bowel and other abdominal viscera protruding from the umbilicus. If the viscera are enclosed in a membrane, conservative measures sometimes give good results, but surgical repair is usually undertaken and is imperative if there is no covering membrane. The term *gastroschisis* describes a more severe and serious congenital defect of the abdominal wall.

2   At later ages

Intestinal obstruction at later ages may be caused by pyloric stenosis, intussusception, volvulus, strangulated inguinal hernia or other rare causes.

Intussusception occurs most commonly in infancy. It has been suggested that the change to a mixed diet leads to a change in intestinal flora and that this causes hypertrophy of Peyer's patches, one of which may form the apex of an intussusception. There is also evidence to suggest that viral infections of the bowel may play a role in causation. The infant cries intermittently with colicky abdominal pain, and between attacks is quiet and pale. The spasms become more frequent and more severe, and distension and vomiting soon develop; red blood may be passed with a rather loose stool ('redcurrant jelly'). Gentle palpation, preferably while the infant is asleep between attacks of pain, will often reveal a firm, sausage-shaped mass lying somewhere in the line of the colon, often in the upper right quadrant. Rarely, the apex may be felt on rectal examination.

A contrast enema not only demonstrates the intussusception but usually leads to its reduction. However, if there is diagnostic delay reduction, at open operation, after correction of fluid and electrolyte balance, may be needed; any gangrenous bowel is resected.

Pyloric stenosis

Congenital pyloric stenosis is a relatively common condition, the cause of which is unknown. The marked preponderance in males (about sevenfold), the increased incidence in twins, and in close relatives, suggest that there is a genetic contribution to the disorder. One the other hand, it is rarely found in stillborn babies, or babies dying within a few days of birth, and it is therefore arguable whether it should be called 'congenital'. The pathology is a hypertrophy of the circular muscle of the pylorus which leads to progressive obstruction. The onset of symptoms is usually gradual, beginning in the second or third week of life, though occasionally much later. Vomiting is initially slight and intermittent but

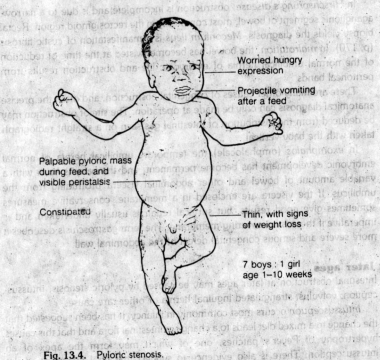

Worried hungry expression

Projectile vomiting after a feed

Palpable pyloric mass during feed, and visible peristalsis

Constipated

Thin, with signs of weight loss

7 boys : 1 girl
age 1–10 weeks

Fig. 13.4. Pyloric stenosis.

becomes more frequent, more copious and more forceful (projectile vomiting). Weight gain, which has usually been satisfactory before the onset of symptoms, falls off, eventually stops, and is followed by weight loss. The motions become more and more constipated. Appetite remains ravenous, but if diagnosis is delayed wasting and dehydration follow (Fig. 13.4). Pyloric stenosis is diagnosed by watching the infant feed; a procedure that may take half an hour. A mass may be felt in the pyloric region before the feed begins, but is often more evident after the feed has been vomited. It is the shape and size of a large olive, very firm, and may be felt contracting intermittently. As the stomach fills, waves of peristalsis become visible, crossing the epigastrium from left to right. Gastric peristalsis increases until the infant vomits, when the vomitus may shoot out several feet. If there is diagnostic difficulty, a contrast meal will show a distended stomach, and a narrow, elongated pyloric canal; ultrasound may demonstrate the enlarged pylorus. The treatment of choice is surgical, the pyloric muscle being divided along its entire length until the mucosa bulges up into the incision (Ramstedt's* operation). Success depends upon adequate pre-operative preparation, skilled surgery and anaesthesia, and careful post-operative management.

INFECTIVE DIARRHOEA

Acute, infective diarrhoea is common: it spreads rapidly through a closed community like a home or a hospital ward, and it is potentially lethal, especially

* Ramstedt and Rammstedt are both correct: he used both.

in the very young or malnourished. The cause may be viral or bacterial, and a similar illness may result from the ingestion of bacterial exotoxins or chemical poisons. Rotaviruses are common pathogens throughout childhood. Bacterial infections are often due to *Helicobacter pylori*. In older children, infections with *Salmonella* and *Shigella* organisms predominate.

In gastroenteritis, diarrhoea and vomiting quickly upset fluid and electrolyte balance. Dehydration causes fretfulness, sunken eyes and fontanelle, and a dry, inelastic skin. Urine output falls; blood urea rises. In some infants water is lost more rapidly than electrolytes causing a rise in serum sodium above 150 mmol/l (*hypernatraemic dehydration*), a condition that may be difficult to diagnose and to treat. In the very young, there may be fever and leucocytosis, suggesting systemic spread of the infection. In these infants, the administration of appropriate antibiotics is probably helpful. In older children with *Salmonella* and *Shigella* infections, antibiotics may delay clearing of the pathogens from the bowel. The basis of treatment is the correction and maintenance of fluid and electrolyte balance. Most can be treated effectively with oral rehydration therapy. The solutions are conveniently made up from pre-packed sachets of dry sugar and salts—glucose accelerates the absorption of solutes from the intestine. Small volumes are given at frequent intervals for a day or two followed by gradual reintroduction of milk. When hospital admission is needed there must be strict barrier nursing to prevent the spread of infection to others. Only a minority require intravenous rehydration.

MALABSORPTION STATES

In children, malabsorption equates closely with steatorrhoea, which is usually due to either coeliac disease or cystic fibrosis of the pancreas. In both conditions the stools are offensive, pale and bulky as well as frequent, and sometimes the mother reports difficulty in flushing them down the toilet because of their tendency to float. Weight gain is unsatisfactory, or there may be frank weight loss with muscle wasting. This contrasts with the big abdomen which is due predominantly to gas and fluid in the distended bowel.

Coeliac disease

Coeliac disease is the result of a sensitivity to the gluten fraction of wheat, rye or other cereals. Therefore symptoms are not to be expected before the introduction of cereals into the diet. There is evidence to suggest that earlier introduction of cereals leads to an increased incidence of coeliac disease—infants do not need cereals before 4 months of age. In addition to the fatty diarrhoea, wasting and abdominal distension, the appetite is usually very poor and the child is miserable. Many of the children have a fair complexion and long eyelashes (Fig. 13.5). The liver is often impalpable. Sometimes the disease begins acutely, and in these children vomiting may be more conspicuous than diarrhoea; indeed, the combination of vomiting and abdominal distension may suggest intestinal obstruction.

There is an enormous range of investigations to which the child suspected of having coeliac disease may be subjected but the diagnosis cannot be made without jejunal biopsy, which shows sub-total villous atrophy on histology. It is mandatory to exclude cystic fibrosis and infection with *Giardia lamblia*.

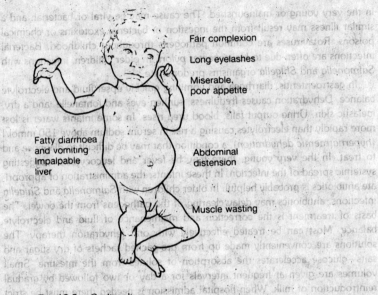

Fair complexion

Long eyelashes

Miserable, poor appetite

Fatty diarrhoea and vomiting

Impalpable liver

Abdominal distension

Muscle wasting

Fig. 13.5.   Coeliac disease.

Treatment consists of exclusion of wheat and rye gluten, and others if necessary. There is usually a rapid and dramatic effect on appetite and temperament, followed by a good weight gain, but some children do not show improvement until they have been on their diet for 3 or 4 weeks. Iron deficiency anaemia is common and as steatorrhoea is associated with deficiency of fat-soluble vitamins, the rapid growth that follows treatment may precipitate rickets. Iron and vitamin supplements are therefore indicated in the early stages of treatment. Although it is often possible for a coeliac child to return to a normal diet in late childhood without a recurrence of diarrhoea, growth may suffer and there is a significant incidence of small bowel lymphoma in adult coeliacs. Strict dietary control for life is therefore advisable. Unfortunately compliance with a gluten-free diet is often poor. Regular follow-up with support from a dietitian is essential. Periodic biopsies at intervals of 2 to 3 years may be helpful in judging compliance. Before committing someone to a life-long gluten-free diet, it is vital to be sure of the diagnosis. As gluten intolerance in early life is occasionally temporary, it is wise to give a gluten challenge followed by a repeat biopsy at a later date.

Cystic fibrosis

Cystic fibrosis is a serious disease that affects about one child in every 2000 amongst white races. In this ethnic group it is the commonest disease caused by an autosomal recessive gene, about 1 person in 23 carrying the gene which causes faulty water and electrolyte transport across cell membranes. The symptoms of the disease, though varied, are largely attributable to the secretion of abnormally viscid mucus. The most helpful laboratory test demonstrates increased concentrations of sodium and chloride in sweat.

Cystic fibrosis may present clinically:

1 As intestinal obstruction in the newborn.
2 As failure to thrive with fatty diarrhoea.
3 With recurrent respiratory infections.

In the newborn baby, the meconium may be so glutinous because of the viscid mucus in it that normal peristalic waves cannot shift it (meconium ileus). Small amounts of meconium may be passed: generalized abdominal distension develops over 24–48 hours, and vomiting develops at the same time. An X-ray of the erect abdomen shows evidence of obstruction. At operation there is often obstruction at several sites, and clearing the viscid meconium may be very difficult. The bowel may have to be opened in several places, and resection may be unavoidable. Unfortunately, even if the obstruction is overcome, the underlying disease remains. Prolapse of the rectum may occur in cystic fibrosis.

If affected infants pass through the neonatal period without illness, they are likely to present later in infancy because of offensive diarrhoea, poor weight gain, respiratory infections, or combinations of these symptoms. Malabsorption is chiefly due to blockage of the pancreatic ducts by viscid secretions and consequent deficiency of pancreatic enzymes. The diarrhoea may start any time from birth, and it is not related to changes in diet. Distension and weight loss resemble those seen in coeliac disease, but the appetite often remains good and the temperament less miserable than in coeliac disease (Fig. 13.6). Recurrent bronchitis and pneumonia (especially staphylococcal) may begin in infancy or may be

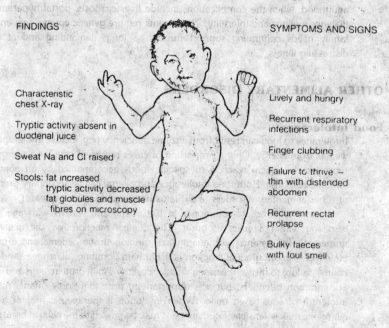

FINDINGS

Characteristic chest X-ray

Tryptic activity absent in duodenal juice

Sweat Na and Cl raised

Stools: fat increased
        tryptic activity decreased
        fat globules and muscle
        fibres on microscopy

SYMPTOMS AND SIGNS

Lively and hungry

Recurrent respiratory infections

Finger clubbing

Failure to thrive — thin with distended abdomen

Recurrent rectal prolapse

Bulky faeces with foul smell

Fig. 13.6. Cystic fibrosis.

delayed for several years. A few children suffer more from sinusitis and nasal polyposis than from chest infections.

Laboratory diagnosis rests chiefly on the demonstration of raised sodium and chloride levels in the sweat (over 60 mmol/l) in the presence of a suggestive clinical picture. Localized sweating is induced by iontophoresis with pilocarpine the sweat is absorbed onto filter paper and analysed chemically. The test is not reliable in very young babies, but thereafter is remarkably specific. (Some mothers notice that the baby tastes salty when kissed). Serum immunoreactive trypsin in blood spots collected at the same time as for phenylketonuria and hypothyroidism is a promising method of neonatal screening. Screening by measuring the protein content of the meconium is associated with an unacceptable number of false negative values in affected infants.

Treatment of the pancreatic disorder consists in the provision of enzymes in powder or tablet form to be taken in adequate doses with food to control the malabsorption. A high energy intake of up to 150% of the usual intake is given together with supplements of fat-soluble vitamins (particularly A, D and E).

The respiratory problems tend to become slowly but progressively worse leading to extensive bronchiectasis and cor pulmonale. Pseudomonas infection is common. The main aim of therapy is therefore the prevention of chest infections and depends upon physiotherapy and chemotherapy. The parents are taught to carry out postural drainage daily and older children taught to do their own physiotherapy. Chemoprophylaxis using antibiotics systemically and/or by inhalation, is used continuously or intermittently, according to circumstances. With modern aggressive therapy started at an early age, most children should reach adulthood, when the complications include liver cirrhosis, portal hypertension, diabetes mellitus and infertility. The parents require genetic counselling; and the family needs continuing support through a long, demanding and at times distressing illness.

OTHER ALIMENTARY DISORDERS

Food intolerance

Intolerance to food can result from enzyme deficiency (e.g. lactose intolerance) as well as from allergy. Only a proportion of cases represent true food allergy, i.e reproducible clinical reaction to specific foods accompanied by an abnormal immune response. Both food intolerance and allergy can be secondary problems of other alimentary disorders (e.g. hiatus hernia and Crohn's disease).

Food intolerance is commoner in the young and lessens with age, most resolving within 3 years of onset. The clinical reaction may be acute and immediate, for instance with anaphylaxis, angioneurotic oedema and urticaria However, a more gradual reaction is usual with vomiting, diarrhoea (and even colitis), failure to thrive or eczema. In infancy, cow's milk protein, eggs and wheat are common offenders, but it is important to note that some infants may be intolerant of soya-based milks. When in doubt, a therapeutic trial of a non allergenic milk is sensible. Food antigens may be passed to the baby in breast milk and cause upset.

After infancy, dairy products and fish are common offenders. Allergy tests are of limited value in diagnosis, although raised levels of IgE specific to individual food proteins are suggestive of allergy. Food additives (e.g. artificial colourings and flavourings) may cause hyperactive behaviour. Trial of a strictly supervised exclusion diet is the best way to make a diagnosis.

Disaccharide intolerance.

Intolerance of disaccharides, notably lactose, may occur:

1 As a temporary complication of gastroenteritis (common).

2 As a temporary complication of coeliac disease or cystic fibrosis (not common).

3 Permanently, as a result of hereditary lactase deficiency (rare).

The condition causes a fermentative diarrhoea. It is diagnosed by demonstrating disaccharides in the stools, which are acid, a positive hydrogen breath test after ingestion of the suspect sugar, and deficiency of disaccharidases in jejunal biopsy specimens. A good clinical response to the exclusion of the offending sugar confirms the diagnosis. If the intolerance is temporary, lactose may be cautiously reintroduced once recovery from the underlying cause is complete.

Note: although children with galactosaemia (p. 220) cannot tolerate lactose, the lesion is not in the alimentary tract and the disease is not usually classified as an intolerance.

Chronic inflammatory bowel disease

Ulcerative colitis and Crohn's disease are not common in childhood and they do not differ in essentials from the adult pattern. Ulcerative colitis most commonly presents with chronic or recurrent bloody diarrhoea with weight loss. Crohn's disease (regional ileitis) most commonly presents with poor growth and obstructive symptoms. In the diagnosis of both conditions, barium enema, colonoscopy and colon biopsy are helpful.

Ulcerative colitis in infants is usually due to cow's milk intolerance and responds to the exclusion of cow's milk. Little else is known of the causes of chronic inflammatory bowel disease, so treatment is empirical and not very satisfactory. Physicians modify the diet (particularly in relation to any associated food intolerance) and prescribe sulphasalazine and steroids; surgeons resect the offending part; neither makes extravagant claims to success.

Acute abdominal pain

Appendicitis occurs at all ages but is uncommon under the age of 2. The most constant features are pain, vomiting, fever and a coated tongue. The diagnosis is usually made on the basis of localized tenderness. With appendix abscess, the history is longer and there is a palpable, tender mass. Diagnostic difficulties may be caused by an appendix in an unusual position, and by other conditions presenting with acute abdominal pain and vomiting. Once an inflamed appendix perforates and peritonitis supervenes, the prognosis becomes worse. If in doubt, 'look and see' is wiser than 'wait and see'.

Toddlers with tonsillitis often compain of pain in the abdomen and not in the throat. Their abdominal tenderness is usually generalized or central, but may be maximal in the right iliac fossa. (Warning: tonsillitis and appendicitis can occur together.)

In acute pyelonephritis the tenderness is usually in the loins. Microscopy and/or culture of the urine gives the diagnosis.

In right lower lobe pneumonia, there may be referred pain and tenderness in the right iliac fossa. The respiratory rate will be raised, there are usually abnormal signs in the chest, and a chest X-ray is helpful.

Mesenteric adenitis is most confidently diagnosed at laparotomy, when enlarged, inflamed glands and normal appendix are found. The condition may be suspected clinically if the child is more tender than ill and if enlarged glands can be felt.

Gastroenteritis often starts with acute abdominal pain and the diarrhoea which makes diagnosis easier may not be apparent for the first 2 or 3 hours.

Hepatic failure

Hepatocellular failure is rare. It may follow fulminating viral infections (e.g. hepatitis, Epstein–Barr), severe obstructive jaundice and a variety of different poisons including paracetamol.

Reye's syndrome is the name given to a devastating illness of young children in which there is an acute encephalitis together with acute liver failure. There is a high mortality and at autopsy the children have fatty degeneration of the liver, kidneys and heart. The cause is unknown but because of a possible association with therapeutic doses of salicylate, aspirin should not be used as an analgesic or antipyretic in children under 12 years.

Giardiasis and worms

Giardia lamblia is a protozoon which commonly inhabits the alimentary canals of children without disturbing their health. Occasionally it causes disease, and this usually takes the form of chronic diarrhoea with semi-formed, khaki-coloured stools and very little constitutional upset. The cysts may be identified in the stools, although their presence does not establish that they are causing disease. Isolation of organisms from duodenal aspirate is more significant. Treatment is with metronidazole.

Threadworms (*Enterobius vermicularis*) are relatively common. They cause no symptoms apart from peri anal itching which may disturb sleep. Diagnosis is made by seeing the worms on the perianal skin or stool, or by demonstrating ova from the peri anal region, best achieved by the use of cellophane swabs or Sellotape. Piperazine is the drug of choice, often given as a single dose combined with standardized senna. Apparent failure is usually due to re-infection. Success is then often achieved by treating the whole family, including parents.

The *roundworm* (*Ascaris lumbricoides*) is uncommon. There are usually no symptoms before a worm is passed with the stools. Piperazine is the drug of choice. *Tapeworms* (*Taenia saginata* and *T. solium*) present with the passage of segments. Treatment may be difficult.

Table 13.3. Causes of rectal bleeding.

Site	Condition	Clinical picture
Ileum	Intussusception	Colicky pain; redcurrant jelly stool; palpable mass
	Bleeding Meckel's diverticulum	Intermittent abdominal pain and bleeding (red or melaena)
Colon	Dysentery (*Shigella, Salmonella*)	Acute mucoid diarrhoea and pain
	Ulcerative colitis	Mucoid diarrhoea: onset sometimes acute
	Intussusception	
Rectum	Polyp	Recurrent bleeding: no pain
	Prolapse	Prolapse visible
Anus	Fissure	On defaecation, much pain and little blood
	Constipation	
	Sexual abuse (buggery)	

Round worm, tape worm and other rarer worms are seen mainly in children returning from developing countries with limited public hygiene.

Rectal bleeding

Blood in the stools is an alarming symptom, although the cause is often trivial. Bleeding from the duodenum or above will usually cause melaena, although copious bleeding (e.g. swallowed blood after epistaxis or tonsillectomy) may cause red blood to appear with the stool. Blood from the ileum or colon is freely mixed with faecal matter; that from the rectum or anus is only on the surface of the stool. If rectal bleeding is associated with painful defaecation, the likely cause is an anal fissure. If a fissure is seen, rectal examination would be very painful and should be avoided.

Many of the important causes of rectal bleeding in adults (e.g. piles, rectal carcinoma) do not occur in children. The main causes in childhood are shown in Table 13.3. Colonoscopy is a helpful investigation particularly for identifying and removing polyps.

Meckel's diverticulum often contains gastric mucosa which may ulcerate and bleed, causing rectal bleeding and anaemia. Radioactive technetium is selectively taken up by gastric mucosa and this provides the basis for an elegant diagnostic test.

FURTHER READING

Jones PG and Woodward AA. *Clinical Paediatric Surgery*. Blackwell Scientific Publications.

Silverman A and Roy CC. *Paediatric Clinical Gastroenterology*. Mosby.

Walker-Smith J Hamilton JR and Walker WA *Practical Paediatric Gastroenterology*. Butterworth.

Chapter 14
Disorders of Bones and Joints

STRUCTURAL VARIATION AND CONGENITAL ABNORMALITIES

The normal flat-footed baby becomes a bow-legged toddler and then a knock-kneed primary schoolchild before growing into a graceful adolescent (Fig. 14.1). Therefore one has to decide whether the source of the parents' concern is normal physiological variation or something requiring further investigation and treatment.

The child should be examined standing and lying in order to detect abnormality of posture, and to check for equal size and length of the limbs. The child should be observed walking or running, and the shoes examined for abnormal wear.

Flat feet

At birth the feet look flat. When children start to stand, at the end of the first year, the feet still look flat because there is a large pad of fat on the soles. The child starts to walk on a wide base with the feet everted and the tibiae externally

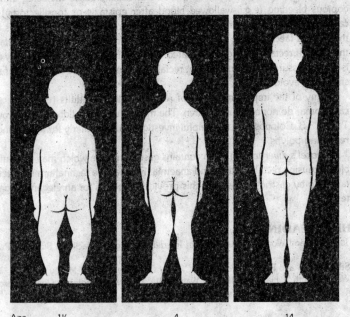

| Age | 1½ | 4 | 14 |

Fig. 14.1. Normal variation of legs with age.

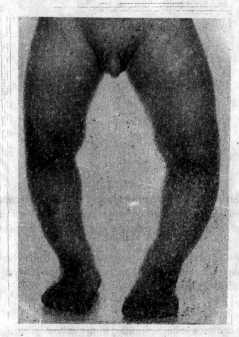

Fig. 14.2. Physiological bow legs in a 1 year old. 2 years later his legs looked straight.

rotated, and the feet still look flat. By the 3rd year the eversion and external rotation have diminished and the feet begin to appear to have a normal plantar arch.

Bow legs (genu varum)
Bow legs are commonest from 0 to 2 years. The knees may be 5 cm apart when the feet are together; the toes point medially (Fig. 14.2). If the degree of bowing is gross, rickets should be excluded (p. 86).

Knock knees (genu valgum)
This is most apparent at 3–4 years of age. When the knees are together, the medial tibial malleoli may be up to 5 cm apart. In obese children the separation may be even greater, but by the age of 12 the legs should be straight. Separation of over 10 cm or unilateral knock knee requires an X-ray, and, probably, a specialist opinion.

Scoliosis
A lateral curve of the spine is commonly seen in babies and may be associated with skull asymmetry. Generally it is a postural scoliosis which goes when the baby is suspended and which has completely gone by the age of 2 years. Scoliosis is again common at adolescence, especially in girls. Asymmetry of scapulae,

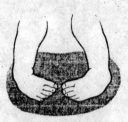
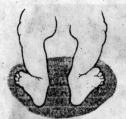

Talipes equino-varus　　　Talipes calcaneo-valgus

Fig. 14.3. Talipes.

shoulders or chest configuration may be more conspicuous than the spinal curve. Usually the spine straightens when it is flexed and eventually corrects itself, but regular review is important because a few progress and require orthopaedic intervention.

Scoliosis may be associated with vertebral anomalies (spina bifida, hemivertebrae) or muscle weakness or imbalance (muscular dystrophy, cerebral palsy), but is idiopathic in 95% of cases.

Talipes (club foot)

Minor degrees of talipes are common at birth, resulting from mechanical pressure *in utero*. The commonest deviation is that in which there is plantar flexion (equinus) and foot adduction (varus) at the midtarsal joint (Fig. 14.3). If the foot with talipes equinovarus can be fully dorsiflexed and everted so that the little toe touches the outside of the leg without undue force, it can be expected to correct itself with time. If it cannot be so overcorrected, urgent splintage or surgery is needed. The sooner treatment is begun the better the outcome. Talipes calcaneovalgus describes the dorsiflexed foot which is everted so that the foot lies against the outer border of the leg with the little toe almost touching it. Usually the position is easily corrected by simple exercises.

Congenital defects of the spinal cord such as spina bifida are commonly associated with severe talipes.

Congenital dislocation of the hip (CDH)

Dislocated hips are associated with joint laxity and acetabular dysplasia. Postural factors play a role in their causation. Congenital dislocation is commoner in:

1　Girls;
2　Babies presenting by the breech;
3　Full-term rather than preterm babies;
4　The left hip.

Diagnosis is made by specifically testing the hips: a modification of Ortolani's manoeuvre is one such test (Fig. 14.4). The baby is laid on its back with the feet towards the examiner. The legs are straightened. Then the examiner grasps the child's legs placing the middle finger of each hand on the outer aspects of each hip, and the thumb on the inner side. In turn each hip is half abducted and the leg is lifted up with the middle finger. A dislocated hip either slips into the socket with

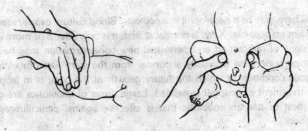

Fig. 14.4. Testing for dislocation of hips.

a click or does not abduct as fully as the normal hip. X-ray examination is unreliable in the first month but ultrasound is increasingly being used for early diagnosis. All babies should be examined in the neonatal period and at intervals during the first year.

One in 60 babies is found to have hip instability (clicking hip) at birth: 85% recover spontaneously, but the remainder persist. Early splinting is successful within 2 months in most neonates. If undetected in the neonatal period, it may not become apparent until the parents worry about their 2-year-old's limp. At that age treatment is more traumatic and less successful.

Osteogenesis imperfecta

This is a group of rare genetic conditions characterized by brittle bones and lax ligaments. In severe cases (usually dominant mutations) muliple fractures occur in utero, whilst milder cases (usually dominant) may merely incur a few fractures between the ages of 4 and 14. Affected children may have blue sclerae and develop deafness in adult life.

Skeletal dysplasias

There are a large number of generalized congenital skeletal dysplasias which are rather rare. Many are genetically determined. The best known is *achondroplasia* (the circus dwarf), due to an autosomal dominant gene but in most cases a new mutation, both parents being normal. There is extreme short stature with disproportionate shortness of limbs, and a large skull vault because of the small skull base. Intelligence is normal.

Several other varieties of short-limbed dwarfism are incompatible with survival after birth. Accurate diagnosis is important for genetic counselling.

OSTEOMYELITIS (osteitis)

Pyogenic infection of bone is commoner in children than adults, and in boys than girls.

The usual site is the metaphysis of one of the long bones, particularly in the legs. At all ages except infancy, *Staphylococcus pyogenes* is the commonest pathogen. The sources of infection and portal of entry are uncertain.

It may present acutely with a high fever and localized pain. An infant may merely refuse to use the affected arm or leg. The cardinal sign of osteomyelitis is a localized point of acute bone tenderness. Over this there may be redness or oedema. There may be a neutrophil leucocytosis. Blood culture usually identifies the organism responsible. X-ray is normal at first: it is only after 2 or more weeks that the signs of rarefaction and periosteal new bone formation may be seen. Radioisotope bone scan is usually abnormal from the start. Osteomyelitis is a most serious condition in which the future growth of the bone is in jeopardy. Intensive treatment in hospital is needed. Large doses of antibiotics are given, and it is best to use an antibiotic that is effective against penicillin-resistant staphylococci.

If treatment is given early, complete resolution occurs in most cases. If diagnosis is delayed surgical drainage is more likely to be needed.

Chronic osteomyelitis may result from inadequate treatment of acute osteo-myelitis or trauma. There is persistent dull bone pain. X-ray shows necrotic areas of bone; it is these areas that harbour the bacteria. Radical surgery to remove necrotic tissue is combined with systemic antibiotics.

ARTHRITIS

Arthritis is characterized by a painful inflamed joint in which there is limitation of movement in all directions. There may be swelling due to fluid in the joint, and redness and heat of the overlying skin. The joint itself is usually painful, but pain arising in the hip may be referred to the knee.

The more important causes are :

1   Those that may result in permanent joint damage:
(a) Juvenile chronic arthritis.
(b) Acute suppurative arthritis due to blood-borne infection. This is treated with aspiration, antibiotics and splintage.
(c) Tuberculosis and brucellosis, now very rare in developed countries.
2   Those that resolve completely (synovitis):
(a) Trauma, especially in schoolchildren. In a child with hip pain and limp ('observation hip') only time may distinguish between trauma and Perthes' disease (p. 182).
(b) Henoch–Schönlein syndrome.
(c) Rheumatic fever.
(d) Serum sickness and generalized allergic reactions.
(e) Viral infections, e.g. rubella (and rubella immunization), mumps and chicken pox causing a 'reactive' arthritis.
Haemarthrosis (bleeding into joints) in children with coagulation disorders may mimic acute arthritis and if recurrent lead to permanent joint damage.

Juvenile chronic arthritis (sometimes called Still's disease)

In young children, this presents with systemic illness—swinging fever, spleno-megaly, lymphadenopathy, erythematous rash—and little or no joint involvement initially. The high ESR and polymorph leucocytosis may suggest infection, and tests for rheumatoid and antinuclear factors are negative.

Older children present with one or more painful, swollen joints and little or no systemic upset. Knees, hips, wrists, ankles and elbows are commonly involved. Neighbouring muscles waste quickly. The term juvenile rheumatoid arthritis is used when the small joints of the hands and feet, the cervical spine and the temporomandibular joints are involved and tests for rheumatoid factor are positive. In juvenile ankylosing spondylitis, the knees and hips are often involved before the spine and sacro-iliac joints, and the children (mostly boys) are usually HLA type B27.

At least 50% of children make a complete recovery, but in others the disease is progressive and crippling. Iridocyclitis is an important complication. Physiotherapy, splintage and the rational use of drugs form the basis of treatment. Non-steroidal anti-inflammatory drugs are appropriate for cases of mild to moderate severity. Penicillamine and gold are used in severe cases but take months to act. Systemic steroids are often necessary.

Other collagen diseases

Systemic lupus erythematosus (SLE), polyarteritis nodosa, dermatomyositis and the other collagen disorders are rare in children. SLE tends to occur in adolescent girls, particularly Blacks. It tends to present as a multisystem disorder; many of the manifestations subside during treatment with corticosteroids, though neurological involvement may be particularly persistent.

Henoch–Schönlein syndrome (anaphylactoid purpura, allergic purpura)

The syndrome is commonest in children aged 2–10 and is made up of a pathognomonic purpuric rash and involvement of one or more of the following: joints, alimentary system and kidneys.

Skin

The rash is distributed over extensor surfaces of the limbs, particularly about the ankles and on the buttocks (Plate 1(a,b)). It begins as a maculopapular red rash, or as an urticarial rash in children under the age of 5, which gradually becomes purpuric (resulting from the vasculitis, the platelet count is normal). Swelling of the face, hands and feet is common and subcutaneous bleeds may occur in the scrotum, eyelids and conjunctivae.

Joints

Pain (arthralgia) of medium-sized joints is common and may progress to an obvious arthritis with red, swollen, tender joints.

Alimentary system

Colicky abdominal pain occurs and may be severe enough to mimic an acute abdominal emergency. Vomiting and diarrhoea are common, haematemesis and melaena less common, and intussusception or perforation very rare.

Kidneys

Microscopic haematuria and transient proteinuria are common. With more severe involvement, the glomerulonephritis causes an acute nephritic syndrome, a nephrotic syndrome or renal insufficiency. The renal complications are responsible for the main morbidity and mortality of Henoch–Schönlein syndrome.

The various groups of symptoms generally present within a week of each other, but may occur in any order and persist for several weeks. Recurrence of any symptoms may occur for several months after onset. The cause is unknown and treatment is symptomatic.

Rheumatic fever (acute rheumatism)

Rheumatic fever is still the most important cause of acquired heart disease in children throughout the world, but in Britain it has become rare. It results from a sensitivity reaction to a group A beta-haemolytic streptococcal infection. Typically there has been acute tonsillitis 1–4 weeks previously.

The child is pale but not always feverish. Nose bleeds are common. The classical pathognomonic features are as follows:

1 *Polyarthritis.* Medium-sized joints are affected—the knees, elbows and ankles. Pain 'flits' from joint to joint as the arthritis affects one joint for a day or two, and then affects another joint.

2 *Carditis.* Tachycardia and a short systolic murmur are usual. More certain evidence of cardiac involvement is a pansystolic or diastolic murmur, a pericardial friction rub or cardiac enlargement leading to cardiac failure. This may resolve or lead to gradual scarring of valves resulting in mitral stenosis and/or aortic incompetence.

3 *Rashes.* Erythema marginatum, a serpiginous red rash with a raised edge found most often on the trunk, is the pathognomonic rash. Erythema nodosum is more common, but not specific.

4 *Subcutaneous nodules,* no bigger than a pea, may be found over bony prominences. They are not tender.

5 *Chorea* (St Vitus' Dance). These involuntary movements are uncommon but may occur in older children up to 6 months after the original streptococcal infection. (This is Sydenham's or rheumatic chorea and is quite different from Huntington's chorea.)

Investigation shows a raised white cell count, and very high ESR (or plasma viscosity) and C-reactive protein levels. Serial antistreptolysin O (ASO) titres show a sustained rise. The ECG may show conduction defects.

It is customary to impose bedrest, particularly if there is heart involvement. Large doses of salicylates are the mainstay of drug treatment though corticosteroids may be used if there is carditis. Anyone who has had rheumatic fever is advised to take daily oral penicillin for life in order to reduce the chance of recurrence.

OSTEOCHONDRITIS AND EPIPHYSITIS

These terms are applied to bone changes that occur, particularly in epiphyses of children, as a result of avascular necrosis.

They present as bone pain, with local swelling and tenderness. There is limitation of movement and adjacent muscle wasting. Those that occur in weight-bearing joints are the most important, as permanent damage may occur. The best example is Perthes' disease which affects the femoral head of children (usually boys) aged 5–8 years. It causes a limp and pain (which may be referred to the knee). The femoral head is softened and will become misshapen if weight-bearing continues, leading to osteoarthritis in early adult life. Treatment

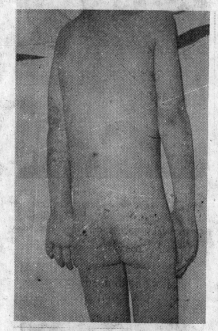

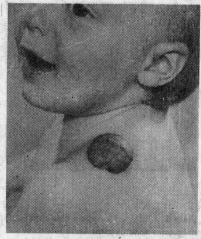

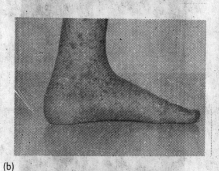

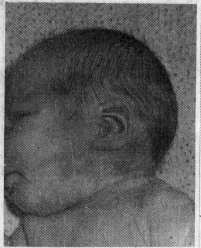

(b)

Plate 1a,b. Henoch–Schönlein purpura. The rash is symmetrically distributed and is most marked over the ankles, buttocks and extensor surfaces.

Plate 3. Portwine stain involving left side of the face. In later life it becomes a much darker colour.

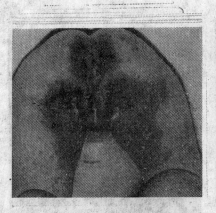

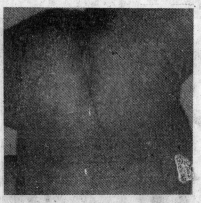

Plate 4. A large Mongolian blue spot with irregular outline over the sacrum with a smaller similar spot over the right upper lumbar region.

Plate 5. Napkin rash—most prominent over the convexities. The involvement of skin creases and pimply margin suggest secondary monilial infection.

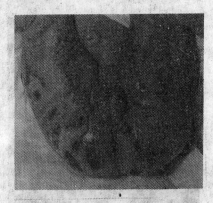

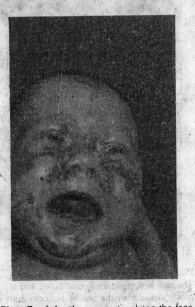

Plate 6. Severe napkin rash with secondary ulceration.

Plate 7. Infantile eczema involving the face and leading to secondary bacterial infection.

with non-weight-bearing calipers allows a reasonably active life until the condition resolves, which may take 2–3 years.

If the affected bone is not a weight-bearing one, the consequences are minimal. Children aged 10–15 are particularly prone to develop transient inflammation of the tuberosity of the tibia (Osgood–Schlatter disease). This resolves satisfactorily without treatment.

FURTHER READING

Cassidy JT. *Textbook of Paediatric Rheumatology*. Wiley Medical.
Hughes GRV. *Connective Tissue Diseases*. Blackwell Scientific Publications.
Sharrard WJ. *Paediatric Orthopaedics and Fractures*. Blackwell Scientific Publications.

Chapter 15
The Skin

Skin disorders are a common reason for children being taken to the doctor. The infant's skin with its thin epidermis and immature glands is particularly liable to infection and blistering. Birthmarks, napkin rashes, infections and eczema are common in pre-school children. Thereafter the incidence of skin disease declines until adolescence when acne is common.

BIRTHMARKS

Birthmarks may involve blood vessels (naevus, haemangioma) or an excess of pigment in the skin. Despite their name, haemangiomata are malformations of blood vessels, not neoplasms. The main types of naevi are:

1 Salmon patch (stork mark)

This is a flat, pinkish capillary haemangioma on the nape of the neck, the eyelids and between the eyebrows (Fig. 15.1). It fades gradually over the first 2 years.

2 Strawberry mark

This is a soft, raised, bright red capillary haemangioma. Sometimes it involves deeper tissues and is combined with cavernous haemangioma which gives it a blue tinge. Common sites are the head, neck and trunk (Plate 2). It is not

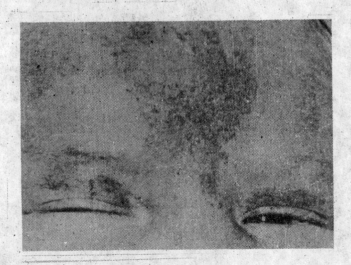

Fig. 15.1 Stork mark. This capillary haemangioma characteristically lies just above the nose, and the upper eyelids are quite commonly affected as in this baby.

apparent until a few days after birth, and usually enlarges during the first 6 months. Thereafter sunken whitish areas develop in the lump and it gradually becomes paler and flatter. Most have disappeared by the age of 7 years. Treatment is best reserved for the very few that are extremely unsightly, do not regress spontaneously, or are expanding rapidly. In general spontaneous regression does not leave a noticeable scar, whilst treatment often does.

3 Port wine stain

Port wine stain is a capillary haemangioma. Since it is flat and, in early life, pale pink it is easily overlooked in the infant (Plate 3) but it darkens to form a flat purple patch of skin which looks ugly. It does not fade. Treatment is difficult. Good results have been achieved using laser, but camouflage with cosmetics is often the best treatment. *Sturge–Weber syndrome* is a rare association of a unilateral port wine stain of the face (including the areas supplied by the divisions of the trigeminal nerve) and an intracranial haemangioma of the pia-arachnoid on the same side. Affected children may present with seizures, hemiplegia, mental handicap or glaucoma.

Abnormal pigmentation

Moles usually develop after the age of 2. They are common and rarely cause anxiety. Single cafe-au-lait spots are without significance, but five or more patches greater than 0.5 cm in diameter suggest neurofibromatosis. Pigmented and de-pigmented lesions are seen in tuberose sclerosis.

Albinism

Albinism consists of a group of genetically determined metabolic disorders characterized by deficient pigmentation. In white people autosomal recessive varieties affect the skin, hair and often the eyes. In black people dominant, partial albinism is more common and does not affect the eyes.

Mongolian blue spots

These are large blue-grey patches, most common over the lumbosacral area and buttocks, which look rather like bruises (Plate 4). They are very common in infants of oriental, Asian or negro stock, but rare in white children. They gradually fade and are rarely visible at the age of 10.

RASHES

Napkin rash

Eruptions of the nakpin area are common in infants. Characteristically, an erythematous rash affects the convexities of the buttocks, inner thighs and genitalia. The skin creases, which do not come into contact with the nappy, are spared (Plate 5). At its simplest it may merely be an irritant rash caused by abrasive napkins or wetness. Fresh urine does not injure the skin, but prolonged contact with stale urine which has broken down to form ammonia products does (ammoniacal dermatitis). In severe cases (Plate 6), papules and vesicles form which ulcerate, leaving a moist surface which easily becomes secondarily infected with either pyogenic organisms or monilia. Secondary infection with monilia usually involves the skin creases. It causes a moist erythematous rash with oval macules and vesicles, a pimply margin and scattered satellite papules.

It is impossible for mothers to change their baby's nappy immediately it is wet. Nappy rashes occur in all classes of society and are not simply confined to babies who have poor care. Some babies have a more sensitive skin than others, and are prone to develop the rash. This must be explained to the mother to dispel needless guilt. However, grossly ulcerated and chronic napkin rashes are a sign of bad care, including infrequent changing.

Treatment is based on the mother carrying out as many of the following instructions as are practicable: frequent and prompt changing of wet nappies including washing and drying the baby's perineum carefully; rubbing a barrier cream or benzalkonium cream on the napkin area; avoiding plastic pants until the rash is cured as these create a hot steamy environment inside; using a 'nappy liner'—a thin specially treated piece of material which transmits moisture to the nappy but remains dry itself. In severe cases the most effective treatment is exposure of the moist rash in a warm dry environment, leaving the nappies off for a few days, together with the use of a dilute hydrocortisone cream to suppress the inflammation. Secondary infection requires local bactericidal or fungicidal cream.

Cradle cap (seborrhoea)

Cradle cap is as common in infants as dandruff and scurf are in older children. It is a thick, light brown crust over the top of the scalp which may look quite difficult to remove. Most chemists sell proprietary brands of medicated shampoo ('cradle cap remover') with which to wash the baby's scalp; alternatively salicylic acid and sulphur cream may be rubbed in before washing the hair. Regular washing of the scalp helps to prevent recurrence.

Some babies develop a more generalized inflammatory skin reaction (seborrhoeic dermatitis) particularly affecting the groins, axillae and neck. Although the skin may be very red and macerated with greasy scaling, it is not irritant and usually resolves within a few weeks. Secondary infection with bacteria or candida may occur.

Eczema

A similar but more troublesome rash is often the first sign of *infantile eczema* (Plate 7). This may be restricted to two or three small lesions or may involve virtually the whole skin surface. Areas commonly involved include the napkin area and the face. Skin cracks behind the pinnae are almost pathognomonic of infantile eczema. The rash is erythematous, scaly or weeping and intensely itchy. Scratching frequently leads to secondary infection (Plate 7). The condition fluctuates, resolves completely in half the children by the age of 2, but in others persists in a mild form or periodically recurs. After infancy the rash is characteristically distributed in the skin flexures, particularly in the antecubital and popliteal fossae (flexural eczema—Fig. 15.2). Prolonged inflammation leads to thick lichenified skin and local lymph gland enlargement.

Frequent bathing in a bath to which emulsifying oil has been added is followed by the local application of steroid ointment or tar paste. Bactericidal creams are

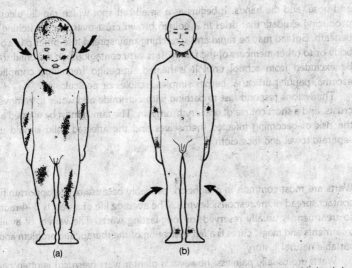

Fig. 15.2 Distribution of eczema: (a) in infancy: cheeks, scalp and behind the ears are commonly affected; (b) in later childhood: skin flexures are affected, particularly antecubital and popliteal fossae.

used for secondary infection. Antihistamines, particularly trimeprazine, subdue the itching. Other measures may include hypnotics at night, and cotton gloves or mittens to limit scratching. The condition tends to improve, and certainly becomes more manageable as the child becomes older.

Environmental factors, including food intolerance, should be considered and for children with severe eczema an exclusion diet is worthy of trial. The child with eczema should avoid contact (particularly kissing) with someone who has herpes simplex (cold sore) because of the risk of developing widespread eczema herpeticum.

Eczema is common in atopic children whose families give a history of asthma, eczema or hay fever. The skin of atopic children is short of protolipids and this predisposes to eczema: the child is also at risk for asthma and hay fever.

Psoriasis

This unpleasant skin condition is commonest at the age of 10–11 and in the early 40s. It tends to run in families and at all ages stress seems to be a provocative factor. The typical lesions are silvery scales on top of a circumscribed salmon-red base. Most types affect principally the extensor surface of the limbs and the scalp; they do not itch. The guttate variety, found mainly on the trunk, appears 2–3 weeks after a streptococcal infection such as tonsillitis. Coal tar ointment and shampoo is the treatment of choice.

Impetigo

This skin infection is usually due to *Staphylococcus aureus* though it is often complicated by streptococcus. It commonly involves the face, around the mouth and nose, and the hands. It begins as a small red spot which rapidly ulcerates, producing exudate that dries in a golden brown crust over the red itching skin beneath. Spread may be rapid and scratching may spread it to other parts of the body or to other members of the family. It is very contagious, so the child should be excluded from school until it is healed. Impetigo frequently complicates ezcema, papular urticaria, herpes simplex, scabies or pediculosis.

The lesions respond fast to bathing with cetrimide and water to remove the crusts, and a short course of oral erythromycin. The family must be warned about the risk of becoming infected themselves and the affected child should use a separate towel and face cloth.

Warts

Warts are most common in childhood, probably because of the opportunity for contact spread of the responsible virus. The average life of a wart is 3–4 months, so treatment is usually reserved for long-lasting warts. The variety of available treatments and magic cures is a fair indication of the therapeutic problem and the variable natural history.

Warts are usually painless; however a plantar wart (verruca) is often painful because the overlying hard skin presses into the foot on walking. Children with plantar warts should be allowed to use swimming baths, but should be advised to cover the wart with a waterproof plaster or wear a covering sock to lessen the chance of transmission.

Urticaria (hives, nettle rash)

Urticaria is common in children, especially under the age of 5. It is characterized by red blotches and whitish weals that itch, and disappear and reappear over a period of hours or days. Sometimes sensitivity to a particular drug or food appears to be responsible.

Oral anti-histamines are effective; adrenaline injection is reserved for severe episodes involving angio-oedema of the face and mouth.

Papular urticaria consists of hard papules most often on the limbs. They appear in crops and itch so that secondary infection is common. In many children, they are associated with insect bites, fleas (including from pets), lice and bed bugs. Papular urticaria tends to recur for a few years each summer.

Erythema nodosum

The shiny red lumps are 1–3 cm in diameter and may be extremely tender. They are most commonly distributed symmetrically over the front of the shins, but do occur elsewhere. During the first week they become more protuberant, purple and painful, then during the next 2 weeks gradually subside and look like old bruises. They may occur at intervals in crops. Although they are thought to represent a hypersensitivity phenomenon to certain stimuli, the provocative stimulus frequently cannot be identified. In childhood, the important associations are:

1 Streptococcal infection.
2 Primary tuberculosis.

3   Certain drugs.
4   Rare diseases such as sarcoidosis, lupus erythematosus and ulcerative colitis.

INFESTATIONS

Pediculosis

The commonest louse infestation in childhood is with the head louse (*Pediculosis capitis*). The louse lives in the hair and lives off blood which it gets by biting the scalp. It causes irritation, and the combination of the bites and the child scratching frequently leads to impetigo and enlarged occipital and cervical lymph glands. The bites may resemble purpura confined to the neck and shoulders. Sometimes the lice can be seen, but more often just the tiny whitish eggs (nits) are seen attached singly to the hair. They can be identified with certainty beneath a microscope: they are ovoid with one blunt end and one pointed end by which they are stuck to the hair shaft. Applications of carbaryl or malathion lotion are rubbed into the hair and left overnight before it is washed. Other members of the home should be examined for similar infestations. (Nits on the eyelashes are likely to represent infestation with pubic lice acquired from an adult).

Scabies

The mite *Sarcoptes scabiei* lays its eggs in burrows beneath the skin. The larva migrates and burrows into the skin, gradually developing into the adult mite, which re-emerges, becomes impregnated and burrows to lay more eggs. After a few weeks the child becomes sensitized and develops a very itchy papulovesicular rash. In older children, this is most marked in the interdigital spaces, wrist flexures and anterior axillary folds. In infants, it frequently involves the face, trunk and feet. The burrows can be seen as small linear elevations of skin adjacent to a small vesicle, but they are often obscured by excoriation and secondary infection. Diagnosis is confirmed by microscopic identification of a mite from one of the burrows. Scabies should be considered as a possible cause for any unexplained itching rash. The infestation is transferred by bodily contact, so that other members of the family are usually affected, and all those living together should be treated at the same time. One or two applications of gamma benzene hexachloride are required and disinfestation of clothing and bedding is advised.

FURTHER READING

Verbov J. *Essential Paediatric Dermatology*. Clinical Press.
Weston WL. *Practical Paediatric Dermatology*. Little, Brown and Co.

Chapter 16
The Urinary Tract

Development

The fetus excretes urine from the 12th week of intrauterine life, and by term it is both swallowing and excreting 500 ml/day. This function is more important for the production of amniotic fluid than for elimination of waste products, since the fetus is being effectively haemodialysed by the placenta.

At birth, renal function is limited. The baby can cope well with normal food intake because body growth is rapid and milk contains exactly the right substances required for growth with little excess. When this situation is altered, the limitations of the immature kidney are seen. If the neonate has excess intravenous fluid, it becomes oedematous. If it has diarrhoea, the kidneys fail to conserve fluid adequately. Compared with the adult a relatively small decrease in renal perfusion, e.g. from mild dehydration or cardiac failure, may result in a raised plasma urea level. This is because the immature kidney has reduced tubular reabsorption, therefore a secondary effect from juxta-medullary feedback (low Cl on the macula densa) is a low glomerular filtration rate. Infants go into renal failure relatively quickly because of this.

Although glomerular function is limited during the first year, it is more efficient than tubular function. Morphologically the glomeruli, which are half adult size at birth, are relatively larger than the tubules. As the kidney matures tubular growth and function increase faster so that by the age of 1 year the adult balance is present. Renal growth continues throughout childhood by means of increase in nephron size, and not by the production of new nephrons. A steady increase of size of renal outline, as assessed by ultrasound or X-rays, is a useful sign of healthy growing kidneys.

The child's kidney is relatively larger than the adult and on X-ray the length should be equivalent to the length of four mid-lumbar vertebrae plus discs.

Urine examination

Routine examination includes inspection, smell, chemical test and microscopy. Careful collection of a fresh specimen, preferably mid-stream, into a clean container is necessary.

1 Inspection

(a) *Translucency*. Fresh urine should appear clear when held up to the light. Chemical deposits are the commonest reason for a cloudy appearance (particularly in cold stale urine); phosphates disappear if 2 drops of dilute acetic acid are added; urates and other acid salts dissolve on gentle warming. Infected urine is usually hazy, and can be frankly cloudy. If the urine is crystal clear, it is unlikely to be infected.

(b) *Colour.* The main influence on colour is the concentration. dilute urine from someone who has drunk a lot being almost colourless. Blood may appear obviously red but more commonly appears pinkish or reddish-brown sometimes with a 'smoky' tint. Ingested foods (e.g. beetroot), confectionery and drugs (e.g. rifampicin) are common reasons for unusual colours.

(c) *Frothiness.* When the container is shaken gently, normal urine settles fast without much froth. Frothiness is a feature of protein or bile in the urine.

2 Smell

In some urine infections, urea-splitting organisms produce a foul fishy smell. This is also the smell of stale urine that has been left standing in a warm place. Some foods and drugs produce characteristic odours (e.g. penicillin). Chemicals produced by body metabolism also influence urine smell: ketones commonly, and products of inborn errors of metalbolism very rarely—because those diseases are extremely rare. (For connoisseurs of smells there is one syndrome that produces a 'sweaty feet' urine, and another that produces 'maple syrup' urine.)

3 Chemical tests

The most convenient are the chemically impregnated test strips ('dipstix'). These should be used according to the directions on the packet. The strip is immersed momentarily in the urine, the surplus urine is dislodged by tapping it and the colour change of the indicator paper is noted at the stipulated time. That time interval is critical for some tests, e.g. haemoglobin. It is important to check that the strip is held the right way round to compare appropriately with the illustrative label on the container.

(a) *Albumin.* A trace of albumin is normal. 5% of children have 1 + (0.3 g/l) or more. Often this is the result of a particularly concentrated sample of urine being tested. If succeeding samples have 1 + or more albuminuria a quantitative estimation must be made. either by estimating the protein–creatinine ratio of a random sample or, more laboriously, collecting a 24-hour sample. Transient albuminuria may occur with fever or hard exercise. Persistent albuminuria is a feature of nephritis and kidney damage.

(b) *Glucose.* Likely causes are a low renal threshold or hyperglycaemia. e.g. diabetes mellitus. (*Clinistix* is specific for glucose. *Clinitest* is a modified Benedict test in tablet form. and detects any reducing sugar.) In the first 2 weeks of life, small amounts of glucose and other reducing sugars are commonly found in the urine.

(c) *Haemoglobin.* Even though the test is extremely sensitive and may be positive when there is no tint of blood on inspection positive reactions are abnormal. The usual cause is haematuria. Since haemoglobinuria and myoglobinuria produce a positive test also. microscopy is mandatory to identify red cells.

(d) *pH.* The usual pH is 5 or 6. Alkaline urine is more likely in infants than in older children because of the frequent feeds: it also occurs after alkaline medicines and sometimes in the presence of urine infection.

(e) *Ketones.* Ketonuria is common in children who are ill. anorexic or have been vomiting, or in the many schoolchildren who have had no breakfast.

4 Microscopy

Regardless of the precise method used, microscopic examination of urine is a most valuable skill. Some people use a counting chamber in order to record the number of formed elements per mm^3 of unspun urine. Others centrifuge the urine and enumerate it (less accurately) per high power field. There is no reliable standard for converting cells per high-power field of centrifuged urine to cells per mm^3 of unspun urine. The urine should be examined under low power with low illumination before increasing the illumination to examine under high power. Constant 'racking' of the fine focus is needed, since the specimen is deeper than a histological specimen.

White blood cells (WBC, pus cells). A healthy boy may have up to 5 WBC/mm^3 and a girl up to $50/mm^3$ (unspun). Excess cells (pyuria) may be the result of a urine infection or inflammation of the renal tract (Fig. 16.1).

Red blood cells (RBC). These may be difficult to identify because they quickly lose their round shape and haemolyse. Urine should not contain more than 2 RBC/mm^3. The commonest causes of haematuria are glomerulonephritis and urinary tract infection. Casts should be searched for to localize the site of the blood loss.

Casts. These are formed in the renal tubules. Cellular casts may be composed of renal tubular cells, but more commonly are composed of red cells, or disintegrating red cells (granular casts). They are an important sign of glomerulonephritis. Hyaline casts devoid of cells are invariably present whenever there is proteinuria, and a few may be present in a concentrated early morning specimen from a normal child.

Bacteria. If the urine is infected bacteria can usually be seen as motile rods, even in unspun unstained urine using the low-power objective. They can be identified more certainly under high power (Fig. 16.2).

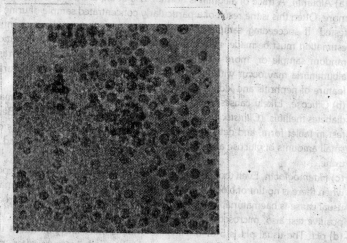

Fig. 16.1   Gross pyuria. The urine contained more than 40 000 WBC/mm, many of them aggregated into clumps. The granular appearance of nucleated white cells is visible on either low- or high-power microscopy.

Fig. 16.2   Bacteriuria. Infected urine viewed under high power: many of the organisms were motile.

CONGENITAL ANOMALIES

Agenesis

This is the result of the ureteric bud failing to develop so that the ureter and kidney are absent. If unilateral. the child may live a full and healthy life provided the other kidney is normal. Bilateral agenesis is lethal. Oligohydramnios has usually been noted during pregnancy. and a proportion of affected infants have a characteristic facial appearance (Potter's syndrome).

Hypoplastic kidneys

The small kidneys are deficient in renal parenchyma. They are not usually associated with other abnormalities.

Dysplastic kidneys

These contain abnormally differentiated parenchyma. They are commonly associated with obstruction and other abnormalities of the urinary tract. *Polycystic disease* represents one form of renal dysplasia. Infantile polycystic disease is associated with massive kidneys. renal failure early in life and a recessive pattern of inheritance. whereas adult polycystic disease which has a dominant inheritance is generally not detected in early life because the kidneys are not enlarged and function well during childhood.

Ureteric abnormalities

Obstruction is commonest at the pelvi-ureteric junction where it may cause hydronephrosis and permanent renal damage. *Duplication* of the ureter and pelvis may occur on one or both sides. If it only affects the upper half of the ureter, it is not important, but if it extends down to the bladder so that there are two separate ureteric openings on that side there are commonly abnormalities of the lower ureter. A *ureterocele* is a cystic enlargement of the ureter within the bladder which may cause obstruction.

Bladder and urethral abnormalities

Posterior urethral valves

These are an important cause of obstruction to urine flow and occur almost exclusively in boys. Bladder neck obstruction is more rare. They usually present in the newborn period or at least in the first year as acute obstruction or chronic partial obstruction with dribbling micturition.

Obstruction of the lower urinary tract is frequently associated with renal dysplasia. But regardless of potential renal function, obstruction may cause direct damage by back pressure or predispose to urinary tract infection which may cause further damage. Most obstructive abnormalities can be corrected by surgery.

Hypospadias

The urethral opening is on the ventral surface of the penis. If it is at the junction of the glans and shaft, no treatment is needed, but if it is on the shaft of the penis plastic surgery is required. The foreskin may be needed for this reconstruction, therefore boys with hypospadias should not be circumcised. In all but the mildest cases, there is ventral flexion *(chordee)* of the penis (Fig. 16.3). There may be associated meatal stenosis.

RENAL DISEASE

Terminology and classification

The starting point for understanding renal disease is to appreciate the classifications that are used.

First, syndromes—collections of symptoms and signs—are defined, e.g. nephrotic syndrome or acute nephritic syndrome.

Second, a pathological or morphological description is given. This is obtained from biopsy or autopsy, e.g. proliferative glomerulonephritis or 'minimal changes'.

Third, an aetiological label is added when this is known, e.g. 'diabetic' or 'post-streptococcal'.

Whilst there are certain correlations between these three levels of diagnosis, it is essential to realize that a particular morphological appearance (for instance, proliferative glomerulonephritis) may be found in each of several different clinical syndromes. Further, a syndrome may be associated with several different morphological pictures, and have several different aetiologies.

The most important syndromes of renal disease in childhood are:

1   Acute nephritic syndrome.
2   Recurrent haematuria.
3   Nephrotic syndrome.

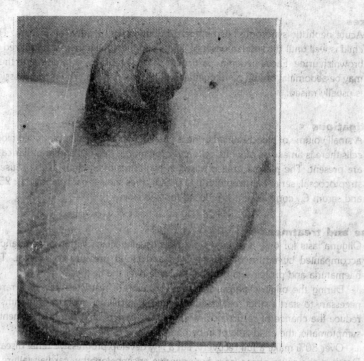

Fig. 16.3 Hypospadias. The meatus is at the junction of the glans and shaft. The prepuce is misshapen and hooded and there is ventral flexion (chordee).

4 Symptomless proteinuria.
5 Urinary tract infection.
6 Renal insufficiency.

ACUTE NEPHRITIC SYNDROME

This is characterized by haematuria, oliguria, hypertension and a raised plasma urea. The last two features are not always present.

Aetiology

The best-known form is post-streptococcal glomerulonephritis, sometimes called acute nephritis. The child has had a beta-haemolytic streptococcal infection, usually a pharyngitis, 2–3 weeks previously. Immune complexes composed of streptococci, antibody and complement are deposited in the glomeruli. There they provoke proliferation of the endothelial cells (proliferative glomerulonephritis). Post-streptococcal glomerulonephritis has become rare in industrialized countries such as Britain, but is common world-wide.

An acute nephritic syndrome may also occur at the time of pneumococcal pneumonia, septicaemia, glandular fever and other viral infections. It is sometimes seen in Henoch–Schönlein syndrome and the collagen diseases.

Features

Acute nephritic syndrome has an age distribution with a peak at 7 years. The child is well until the sudden onset of illness and the appearance of bright red or brownish urine. Facial oedema, particularly of the eyelids, is common, and there may be abdominal or loin pain together with loin tenderness. The blood pressure is usually raised.

Investigations

A small volume of blood-stained urine is passed. In addition to copious red blood cells there is an excess of white cells and proteinuria. Red cell and granular casts are present. The plasma urea is raised in two-thirds of children. If the cause is streptococcal, serial antistreptolysin O (ASO) titres show a rise to above 1 : 250, and serum C_3 complement is reduced for 2–8 weeks.

Course and treatment

Oliguria lasts for only a few days. Diuresis usually occurs within a week and is accompanied by return of plasma urea and blood pressure to normal. The haematuria and proteinuria gradually subside over the next year.

During the oliguric phase, fluid and protein are restricted, but it is rarely necessary to start a strict renal failure regime. Penicillin is given for 3 months to reduce the chance of recurrence, which in any case is rare. Other treatment is symptomatic; the child is kept in bed only as long as he feels ill.

Over 80% make a full recovery, but a few develop progressive renal disease. Death in the acute phase from hypertensive encephalopathy, cardiac failure or acute renal failure is very rare.

RECURRENT HAEMATURIA SYNDROME

This is characterized by recurrent bouts of haematuria, which may occur at the time of a systemic infection or exertion. The child may feel mildly unwell but more often has no symptoms. The haematuria results from nephritis of unknown cause.

Between attacks the urine is normal or shows microscopic haematuria. Proteinuria is less common and may indicate more serious renal disease.

Investigations are done to exclude other causes of haematuria: urine culture, ultrasound scan and X-ray for a tumour or stone, and screening tests for bleeding disorders. If, as is usual, the urine contains red cell and granular casts, cystoscopy constitutes an improper assault, since casts originate from the kidneys.

A small minority have serious and progressive nephritis, but the majority have a good prognosis. Their renal function is normal and continues so.

The bouts of haematuria may continue for several years, and the doctor who has the task of reassuring the parents usually ends up wishing that blood was colourless. Prolonged restriction of activity or bedrest is more likely to result in an uneducated delinquent adolescent than to affect the renal prognosis.

NEPHROTIC SYNDROME

Nephrotic syndrome is characterized by heavy proteinuria, hypo-albuminaemia and oedema.

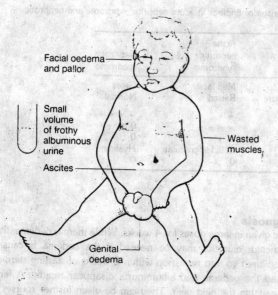

Facial oedema
and pallor

Small
volume
of frothy
albuminous
urine

Ascites

Wasted
muscles

Genital
oedema

Fig. 16.4 Nephrotic syndrome.

Features

Peak onset is between the ages of 2 and 5 years. Apart from the gradual onset of generalized oedema, the child may be only mildly off colour. Other symptoms are directly related to oedema, for instance discomfort from ascites or breathlessness from pleural effusion (Fig. 16.4).

Aetiology

Over 90% of childhood nephrotic syndrome is the result of primary renal disease of unknown cause. Nephrotic syndrome secondary to systemic illness is less common than in adults, the least rare causes being Henoch–Schönlein syndrome and the collagen diseases. In Africa, quartan malaria is an important cause.

Pathology

Up to the age of 5 years, over 80% of affected children will show only 'minimal changes'. This means that the biopsy reveals no significant abnormality on light microscopy, immunofluorescence or electron microscopy. After the age of 10, more serious pathology becomes likely.

Investigations

The urine is frothy and there is heavy albuminuria. Highly selective proteinuria, that is urine containing a high proportion of small molecular weight proteins, is a good prognostic feature suggesting minimal change histology. Hyaline casts are abundant (see Table 16.1). Serum albumin is below 25 g/l and the serum cholesterol is usually raised. Plasma urea is usually normal.

Table 16.1. Comparison of findings in acute nephritic syndrome and nephrotic syndrome.

		Acute nephritic syndrome	Nephrotic syndrome
Child:	Oedema	Mild-facial	Gross
	Blood pressure	Raised	Normal
Urine:	Albumin	+ +	+ + + +
	RBC	+ + + +	0 or +
	WBC	+ +	0
	Casts	Cellular/granular	Hyaline
	Bacteria	0	0

Treatment and prognosis

Corticosteroids are given in large doses for 4 weeks. While there is oedema, fluid and salt are restricted: diuretics may be needed if the oedema is causing symptoms. Most children go into remission within 2 weeks of starting steroids. Diuresis occurs and the oedema and albuminuria disappear rapidly. A large proportion relapse within the next year. They can be given further courses of steroids, but if the relapses are frequent cyclophosphamide will usually produce a longer remission.

The long-term prognosis is good. Although frequent relapses can be most troublesome during childhood, with increasing age they become less frequent and most children 'grow out' of the condition by the time they are adults and thereafter retain normal renal function and good health. A few (mainly those initially unresponsive to steriods) develop renal insufficiency. Unusual features at onset which are unfavourable prognostic signs are: late age of onset, haematuria, hypertension or raised plasma urea. Renal biopsy tends to be reserved for children showing these features.

SYMPTOMLESS PROTEINURIA

Persistent proteinuria with a urinary excretion of more than 0.3 g/day is abnormal (see p. 191). It may be a sign of renal disease and requires investigation. Before embarking on elaborate tests of renal function or a biopsy, it is important to exclude postural (orthostatic) proteinuria, since this is commonest in the age range 10–15 years. Such children do not have proteinuria when recumbent in bed, but have excess proteinuria when up and active, particularly after adopting an excessively lordotic position. Postural proteinuria is generally considered a benign condition which does not progress.

URINARY TRACT INFECTION

Infection of the urinary tract is one of the commonest and most puzzling conditions of childhood. Because it is unusual to be able to localize the infection to any particular site, it is preferable to call it 'urinary tract infection' than to use words such as 'cystitis' or 'pyelitis'.

Incidence

From birth to adolescence the prevalence of urinary tract infection is just over 1%. In the neonatal period, boys are more often infected, but thereafter girls predominate. By the age of 2 years, 5% of girls have had a urinary tract infection, and during the school years infection is 25 times more likely in a girl.

Pathology

The commonest pathogen is *Escherichia coli*. Bacteria of the same strain are usually present in the child's gut and it is assumed that the organism enters the urethra via the perineum.

Features

The child may have neither symptoms nor signs. When there are symptoms they tend to be non-specific: feeding problems, fever, prolonged jaundice in the neonate; vague malaise, enuresis or urgency in the older child. The classic adult picture of burning dysuria, fever and loin pain is less common.

Investigations

The diagnosis is made if a carefully collected clean specimen of urine contains more than 10^8 organisms/l in pure growth. A mixed growth is more likely to be the result of contamination than infection. A culture yielding less than 10^7/l is normal, a count in between means that the culture must be repeated. The greatest problem in infants is obtaining a clean urine sample. Self-adhesive perineal plastic bags are widely used; they must be emptied immediately urine has been passed to avoid perineal contamination. Children's wards sometimes use wet (or warm)-sensitive electronic devices for notifying the nurses as soon as micturition occurs. Such 'squirt-alerts' or 'pee-peepers' allow fresh urine to be collected and despatched promptly for culture. Occasionally it is necessary to resort to supra-pubic aspiration of urine directly from the bladder using a syringe and needle. The infant's bladder lies relatively higher above the pubis so that it is not difficult to aspirate.

Macroscopically, the urine may have an opalescent sheen. Microscopically, bacteria are seen (usually motile rods) and there may be an excess of white cells. The presence of albuminuria is irrelevant to diagnosis. Haematuria may be present.

Management

1 *Initial treatment.* Fluid intake is increased and frequent micturition encouraged. Appropriate chemotherapy is given: nitrofurantoin or trimethoprim are used widely. There is increasing evidence that a 1-day course (or even just 1 large dose) is as effective as a longer course for uncomplicated infections.

2 *Further investigation.* Ideally an ultrasound scan and abdominal X-ray should be done on any child who has had a definite urinary infection. The aim is to detect obstructive abnormalities. This is followed by further radiology if necessary. Vesico-ureteric reflux is present in a quarter of children with urine infection, but minor degrees of reflux in which a wisp of urine is seen to pass through the lower part of the ureter are unimportant. When there is major reflux, the urine refluxes

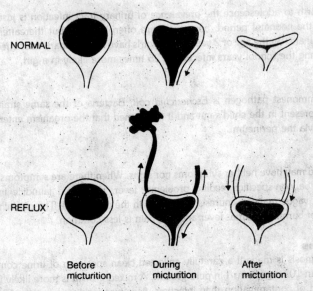

NORMAL

REFLUX

Before
micturition

During
micturition

After
micturition

Fig. 16.5 Vesico-ureteric reflux (shown by micturating cystogram). At the end of micturition there remains in the bladder a puddle of stagnant urine.

up the ureter filling and distending the calyces, and at the end of micturition falls back to form a stagnant pool (Fig. 16.5). Reflux is commoner in children than in adults, and, providing recurrent infections can be prevented, for instance by prophylactic antibiotics, it tends to go as the child grows. If medical treatment is unsuccessful, surgical correction of the reflux is possible.

3 *Follow-up* is an important part of the management. One-third of children will have a recurrence within the next year. The child's urine must be cultured a few days after completing the initial therapy and at least once in the next 3 months, *even though the child is symptomless.*

The problem of prognosis

Infection of the renal parenchyma may cause permanent or progressive damage leading to renal insufficiency. Although radiologists sometimes describe such small scarred kidneys as 'chronic pyelonephritis', a truer morphological label is chronic interstitial nephritis. The same morphological appearance is seen in the later stages of renal disease of many origins other than infection. It is clear that the vast majority of the multitude of children with urinary tract infection do not incur renal damage. Renal damage is most likely in those with associated obstruction of the urinary tract, and in those who have severe infection and gross reflux early in life—under the age of 2. For the vast number of girls who have recurrent infections with or without symptoms during their school days serious renal damage is unlikely. It is sufficiently rare for some experts to suggest that treatment of symptomless urine infection is not necessary.

RENAL CALCULI

Stones in the urinary tract of children are less common than in adults. Occasionally they cause pain or renal colic but more often are detected by chance on X-ray. Most stones are of infective origin, especially in boys with a proteus infection. Since they can be of metabolic origin it is customary to check the urine for abnormal amino acids (e.g. cystinuria) and the serum calcium and phosphate.

RENAL INSUFFICIENCY (renal failure)

Acute renal failure describes the situation in which previously healthy kidneys suddenly stop working. It is a rewarding condition to treat in childhood because a higher proportion of children have recoverable conditions than do adults who present acutely.

A particularly notorious form is the *haemolytic–uraemic syndrome* which affects mainly older infants and toddlers. After a brief gastroenteritis–like illness the child presents with a haemolytic anaemia, thrombocytopenia and acute renal failure. Early peritoneal dialysis and expert management in a paediatric renal unit enable more than 80% to recover completely.

Progressive renal insufficiency or chronic renal failure is uncommon. During the early months of life, congenital abnormalities, particularly renal dysplasia, are the main cause. Thereafter various forms of glomerulonephritis are the commonest cause. Children with end-stage renal disease have the same features as adults, e.g. anaemia, hypertension and renal rickets; in addition they fail to grow.

Successful transplantation is the aim, and results for children are better than for adults. Until transplantation is possible the child is maintained on dialysis; continuous/intermittent ambulatory peritoneal dialysis is frequently used despite the common complication of peritonitis.

THE GENITALIA

Undescended testicles

The testicles normally descend into the scrotum about the 36th week of gestation and are therefore usually fully descended in the newborn full-term infant. Spontaneous descent may occur later, but the older the child the less likely is this to happen. If a testis remains undescended until after puberty, it will not mature properly and will be sterile. 'Undescended' testicles are often incompletely descended and are palpable in the inguinal canal. If such a testis cannot be persuaded into the scrotum, or if the testis cannot be felt at all, orchidopexy is advised.

Incompletely descended testes need to be distinguished from retractile testes and ectopic testes. Retractile testes are very common and normal. An active cremaster muscle will withdraw the testis into the inguinal canal or higher, especially if the doctor has cold hands. Ectopic testes are rare and may be located in the superficial inguinal pouch, near the femoral ring, or in the perineum.

Hydrocele

At birth it is quite common to find fluid in the scrotal sac. It almost always clears up without treatment. In older infants and children there may be a tense hydrocele on one or both sides. It does not cause symptoms but is often associated with inguinal hernia. Surgery is therefore advised.

Circumcision

The foreskin is normally adherent to the glans in the early months of life and sometimes for as long as 3 or 4 years. In infancy, therefore, the foreskin can only be retracted by breaking down the adhesions, a procedure that is unnecessary for the baby and distressing for the parents. A non-retractile prepuce in early life is not an indication for circumcision. If the preputial orifice is small enough to obstruct urine flow (phimosis), circumcision is indicated. Paraphimosis is usually treated by an emergency dorsal slit followed later by circumcision.

Posthitis (inflammation of the foreskin) is common in babies while they are still in nappies. It requires treating as for nappy rash and is a contraindication to circumcision because of the risk of a meatal ulcer. If normal separation of the foreskin from the glans does not occur by about the third year of life, or if the foreskin cannot be retracted in order to clean underneath, then balanitis (inflammation of the glans) may occur and may be an indication for circumcision.

Hypospadias is a contraindication to circumcision because the foreskin is used by the surgeon to fashion an anterior urethra. Jews and Muslims require their boys to be circumcised.

Adherent labia minora

Sometimes firm adhesions develop between opposing surfaces of the labia minora (Fig. 16.6), probably as a consequence of poor personal hygiene. Urine is passed normally, but the appearance may suggest that there is no vaginal orifice. The labia may be separated with a probe or repeated application of oestrogen cream.

When having their perineum examined, young girls are likely to be happiest if lying supine on their mother's lap or on a couch with their legs up in the lithotomy position. They can see what the examiner is up to. The labia are gently pulled apart to check that they are not adherent and the vulva is inspected. Vaginal examination is a little more difficult. If the child crouches forward in the prone position with the chest well down, the knees slightly apart, and the bottom stuck in the air this tends to open the vagina and inspection can be done using a torch and without the need to put anything in the vagina.

Vaginal discharge

Soreness and irritation of the vulva in girls is usually due to lack of personal hygiene. Micturition may be painful. Staining of the pants may result from normal heavy secretion of mucus particularly about puberty. Careful daily washing and drying of the perineum will relieve both conditions. A purulent vaginal discharge is less common.

Pus should be cultured and examined for *Trichomonas* and other sexually transmitted disease. The possibility of sexual abuse or an underlying foreign body should be borne in mind.

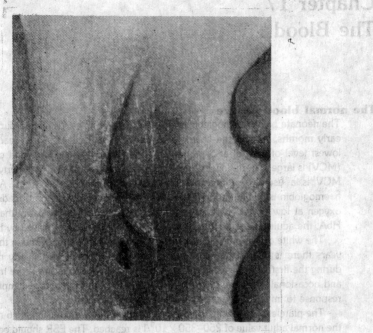

Fig. 16.6 Adherent labia. The labia are adherent throughout most of their length but a small orifice remains through which urine is passed. N.B. This orifice is not the vagina.

The causes of *vaginal discharge* are summarized below:

1 White mucoid (leucorrhoea):
   (a) in neonate. normal:
   (b) at puberty. normal.
2 Offensive yellow (vulvovaginitis):
   (a) aged 2–5. associated with poor hygiene:
   (b) infection:
   (c) sexual abuse:
   (d) foreign body.
3 Bloody (vaginal bleeding):
   (a) in neonate may be normal:
   (b) sexual abuse:
   (c) foreign body:
   (d) tumour:
   (e) menarche.

FURTHER READING

Edelmann CM, Bernstein J. Meadow SR and Spitzer A. *Paediatric Kidney Disease*. Little. Brown and Co.

Postlethwaite RJ. *Clinical Paediatric Nephrology*. Wright.

Williams I and Johnston J. *Paediatric Urology*. Butterworth.

Chapter 17
The Blood

The normal blood picture

The neonate has a haemoglobin of 19 g/dl. Erythropoiesis is limited during the early months, so that the haemoglobin level falls (Table 17.1). It reaches its lowest level of 11 g/dl at 3 months and thereafter rises steadily. Red cell size (MCV) is large at birth, low at 1 year and rises to the adult level at puberty; a low MCV is a useful sign of iron deficiency or of thalassaemia trait. At birth haemoglobin is mainly of the fetal type—HbF. This combines more readily with oxygen at low oxygen tensions, and also gives up CO_2 more easily than does HbA, the adult type. During the first year HbF is gradually replaced by HbA.

The white cell count is relatively high throughout childhood, and in the early years there is a preponderance of lymphocytes which is particularly marked during the first year. Leucocytosis in response to infection is also more marked, and occasionally includes a few primitive white cells. In infants, a lymphocytic response to infection does not exclude a bacterial cause.

The platelet count is slightly reduced in the first few months but by 6 months the normal adult value of $250–350 \times 10^9/l$ is reached. The ESR should be below 16 in childhood, provided that the packed cell volume is at least 35%. Plasma viscosity is a satisfactory alternative to ESR.

ANAEMIA

Anaemia is common in childhood, but not quite as common as many mothers suspect. Mothers are often worried by their child's pallor, which is more often a feature of a fair complexion than of anaemia. Anaemia may cause tiredness and even breathlessness, but most tired children are not anaemic. Examination of the mucous membranes is more reliable than skin colour, but whenever anaemia is suspected a blood test is necessary.

Anaemia may be caused by:

1 Diminished production of red cells.
2 Excessive breakdown of red cells.
3 Blood loss.

Table 17.1. Normal blood picture.

Age	Haemoglobin		MCV	WBC ($\times 10^9/l$)	Lymphocytes (%)
	(g/dl)	Type			
1–2 weeks	18	HbF>HbA	96	12.0	70
1 month	15	HbF>HbA	91	11.0	65
3 months	11	HbF<HbA	84	11.0	65
1 year	12	HbA	78	10.0	55
4 years	13	HbA	80	9.0	40
12 years	14	HbA	81	8.0	30

1   Diminished production

(a) Deficiency anaemias

Iron deficiency anaemia is by far the most common, and is characterized by a hypochromic microcytic blood picture (Fig. 17.1). Reduction in MCV is a useful early sign, and is followed by a reduction of mean corpuscular haemoglobin concentration to less than 32 g/dl. Basically it is caused by insufficient intake of iron, which is more common in the following groups of children:

(i) Preterm babies and twins (p. 66).

(ii) Infants who have to exist entirely on milk and are late changing to iron-containing weaning foods—sometimes because the infant is retarded or has cerebral palsy and is late learning to chew solids.

(iii) Children from homes where poverty, ignorance, or religious/racial factors prevent the child from receiving red meat, green vegetables, eggs, and bread (which are the main sources of iron). Older infants and toddlers are most at risk.

(iv) Children with chronic malabsorption who fail to absorb iron.

(v) Adolescent girls who are undergoing a phase of rapid growth at a time when they are also losing blood from menstruation.

Other deficiency anaemias are uncommon. Folic acid deficiency in British children may be seen in malabsorption syndromes. Pernicious anaemia is extremely rare in children. Hypothyroidism and scurvy are associated with hypochromic anaemias which are corrected by treatment of the primary conditions.

(b) Bone marrow disturbance

Infiltration. Leukaemia (p. 211) is the most important infiltrative disturbance which may present as anaemia. Secondary deposits from malignant tumours and lipidoses are less common.

(c) Toxic damage

Chronic infection and renal insufficiency depress haemopoiesis. Many toxins, including drugs, can suppress marrow activity and cause *aplastic anaemia*.

2   Excessive breakdown

Haemolytic anaemias are not as common as deficiency anaemias, but are important as some are specific to children and others cause their main problems in childhood. They are characterized by chronic or recurrent normochromic anaemia with slight jaundice at times. While haemolysis is active, there is usually a reticulocytosis, but there is sometimes marrow aplasia at the time of acute haemolysis. When the haemolysis is severe and sudden, it is called a 'haemolytic crisis'; jaundice, dark urine and dark stools are likely. Splenomegaly is a feature of chronic cases. Haemolysis results from abnormalities of the red blood cells or abnormal factors in the plasma.

(a) Cellular abnormalities

These comprise abnormalities of red cell shape, intracellular enzymes, or haemoglobin structure.

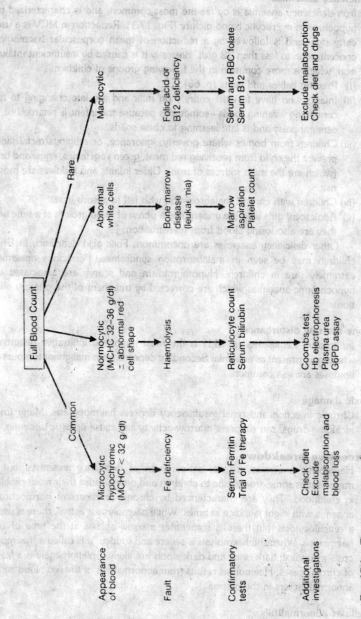

Fig. 17.1. The investigation of anaemia.

(i) *Red cell shape.* The most important abnormality is *hereditary spherocytosis* (acholuric jaundice) in which the red cells are small and spherical and show increased osmotic fragility. It is inherited as a dominant characteristic, but one-third of cases are new mutations.

(ii) *Enzyme defect.* The commonest is *glucose-6-phosphate dehydrogenase* (G6PD) *deficiency.* It is rare in Britain except in persons of Mediterranean, African or Chinese origin. X-linked recessive inheritance occurs. Affected boys often develop neonatal jaundice, and are susceptible to certain chemicals, such as primaquine, aniline derivatives and PAS. Some of the children develop haemolysis after eating the Fava bean (a type of broad bean) or inhaling the pollen of the flower; this is called favism.

(iii) *Haemoglobinopathies.* The synthesis of haemoglobin is under genetic control. Some abnormal genes interfere with the production of entire globin chains (e.g. β chains) so that the affected person lacks normal haemoglobin (e.g. β thalassaemia). Other abnormal genes result in the substitution of an amino acid in the globin chain, so producing an abnormal haemoglobin (e.g. HbS). These two examples are the most important haemoglobinopathies.

Children with *thalassaemia* have a persistent preponderance of HbF and a deficiency of HbA. It is inherited as an autosomal recessive trait, and occurs in a broad belt extending from the Mediterranean countries through India to the Far East. The Mediterranean form is usually β thalassaemia; α thalassaemia, which causes hydrops and perinatal death, occurs mainly in the Far East. In the UK most affected people have originated from Cyprus, the Middle East or the Indian subcontinent. Those with the heterozygous state have thalassaemia trait and are asymptomatic or have a mild anaemia. Their red cells contain up to 20% HbF. Those with the homozygous state have more profound anaemia, the Hb level depending upon the balance of red cell production and destruction. Sometimes an acceptable level is sustained (thalassaemia intermedia) for a while, but later falls (thalassaemia major). There is active extra-medullary haemopoiesis, with hepatosplenomegaly, and hyperplasia of bone marrow which involves the cranial bones and leads to a characteristic facial appearance unless prevented by treatment.

Treatment involves regular blood transfusion every 3–4 weeks to maintain a high Hb level, desferrioxamine by nightly subcutaneous infusion to prevent iron overload, and supplements of folic acid and vitamin C to support red cell production. Hypersplenism may develop. Prenatal diagnosis and carrier detection are well-established, using DNA probes.

Sickle-cell disease occurs in the Negro races. HbS is present in place of HbA. At low oxygen tensions the cell becomes crescent or sickle-shaped and is likely to haemolyse. The heterozygotes have about 30% HbS, may show sickling, but are usually symptomless. The homozygotes develop recurrent episodes of haemolysis during infancy. In addition to the problems of haemolytic and aplastic episodes that occur in any haemolytic anaemia, those with sickle-cell disease also may develop intravascular thromboses. Most commonly thromboses occur in mesenteric, intracranial or bone vessels. The symptoms simulate acute abdominal emergencies, meningitis or arthritis. Treatment is symptomatic, and the prognosis poor; many die in late childhood or early adult life from infections, cardiac failure, or thrombotic episodes. However, the outlook is better if the general health and nutrition of the child is improved. DNA probes are available for prenatal diagnosis and carrier detection.

(b) Extracellular abnormalities

Antibodies causing premature destruction of the red cell are usually associated with a positive Coombs' test. The only common example in childhood is haemolytic disease of the newborn (p.74). Rarer causes include severe poisoning or infection, malignancy and systemic lupus erythematosus.

3   Blood loss

Hidden blood loss is not common in childhood, peptic ulcers, piles and gastro-intestinal malignancy being rare. Gastrointestinal bleeding from a Meckel's diverticulum or reflux oesophagitis is more likely to present with overt bleeding than unexplained anaemia.

COAGULATION DISORDERS

Haemophilia

Most cases (haemophilia A) are caused by deficiency of plasma Factor VIII. A minority are caused by deficiency of Factor IX (Christmas disease or haemophilia B). Both are caused by X-linked recessive genes, so that on average half the sons of female carriers are affected. The condition usually presents during the second year of life with excessive bruising as the child learns to crawl and walk. Alternatively there is prolonged bleeding following circumcision, blood sampling or tooth eruption.

Haemarthroses, especially of the ankles and knees, are one of the major problems of haemophilia: recurrent haemarthrosis can lead to permanent joint damage and chronic disability. The blood shows a prolonged clotting time and partial thromboplastin time; specific assay of the relevant coagulation factors is then performed to identify the precise abnormality.

Severity is related to the degree of deficiency of the relevant factor. Just under half have less than 1% of normal factor activity and can be classified as 'severe'. Those with over 5% of activity have 'mild' haemophilia and experience problems only after obvious injury or surgery.

Treatment of bleeding episodes consists of the intravenous injection of concentrates of the deficient factor. Many families manage their own injections. There are risks of hepatitis B (immunization is important). Unfortunately the blood products used in the treatment of haemophilia in the 1970s and early 1980s were often contaminated with HIV. More than half of those with haemophilia treated before 1985 are now HIV positive. Modern concentrates are heat-treated to prevent HIV transmission.

Haemarthroses require careful orthopaedic management. One of the most difficult problems is to protect the child from trauma, by forbidding certain activities, and yet allowing him to lead an enjoyable and profitable life. Regular prophylactic dental care is important. Haemorrhage after dental extraction and other surgical procedures can be avoided by admitting the child to hospital for factor replacement. Haemophilia usually becomes less severe as adult life is reached. Regional haemophilia centres provide skilled, coordinated care. One of their functions is to provide a service for the identification of female carriers. Prenatal diagnosis is possible.

Von Willebrand's syndrome affects both boys and girls. Though there is a combination of Factor VIII deficiency and platelet dysfunction, the degree of the bleeding disorder is usually mild.

Thrombocytopenia

Thrombocytopenia may be a feature of several systemic diseases as well as infiltrative diseases of the bone marrow and marrow aplasia. However, the most common thrombocytopenic purpura of childhood is *idiopathic thrombocytopenic purpura* (ITP). The onset is acute, often occurring 1–3 weeks after an upper respiratory tract infection. A widespread petechial rash appears, developing into small purpuric spots (purpuric spots do not fade when pressed). There may be bleeding from the nose or into the mucous membranes. There are no other abnormal signs, and the haemoglobin and white cell count are normal. The platelet count is very low, usually below $30 \times 10^9/l$. The bone marrow often shows an *excess* of immature megakaryocytes.

Generally the outcome is good. Seventy-five percent of children have made a complete recovery within one month of onset and have no further trouble. Transfusions of platelets and blood may be needed at onset. Corticosteroids in large doses reduce the risk of massive haemorrhage and accelerate the natural recovery in most children. Splenectomy is reserved for the small minority who have persistent or recurrent thrombocytopenia. Other causes of purpura are shown in Table 17.2.

Disseminated intravascular coagulation
(DIC, consumption coagulopathy)

This syndrome is an important cause of bleeding and purpura. It is convenient (though an oversimplification) to consider that intravascular coagulation uses up platelets and other factors, causing overt bleeding elsewhere; and that as the circulating blood is forced through the intravascular clots some of the red cells are damaged, become fragmented and haemolyse. There is bleeding and purpura. Examination of the blood shows haemolytic anaemia, fragmented red cells, thrombocytopenia and deficiency of coagulation factors. In the neonate, it occurs as a result of severe anoxia or massive infection. In older children, it may be associated with septicaemia, cyanotic congenital heart disease and vasculitis. The prognosis is grave but recovery is possible.

Table 17.2. The main causes of purpura in childhood.

Platelet count low (thrombocytopenia)	Platelet count normal
Idiopathic thrombocytopenic purpura	Henoch–Schönlein syndrome (p. 181)
Leukaemia (p. 211)	Septicaemia (particularly meningococcal)
Toxic effect of drugs	Common infectious illnesses and viraemia

FURTHER READING

Modell B and Berdonkas V *The Clinical Approach to Thalassaemia*. Grune and Stratton.

Miller D, Baehner R and McMillan C. *Blood Diseases of Infancy and Childhood*. CV Mosby.

Willoughby MLN. *Paediatric Haematology*. Churchill Livingstone.

Chapter 18
Neoplastic Disease

Malignant disease is the second most frequent cause of death between the ages of 1 and 15 years. Accidents are the commonest cause of death. Although malignancy is an important cause of death, it is nevertheless uncommon—only 1200 newly diagnosed cases occur in the UK annually out of a childhood population of 12.5 million.

Malignancy is not only less common than in adults, it is also different in origin and course. The epithelial malignancies of adult life, carcinomata of respiratory, gastrointestinal and reproductive tracts, are rarely seen in childhood. The commonest malignancies of childhood are those of the reticuloendothelial system: leukaemia and lymphoma. These are followed in order of frequency by brain tumours and then by primitive blast cell tumours and sarcomata of the kidney (Wilms' tumour), adrenal (neuroblastoma) and muscle tissue (rhabdomyosarcoma). Childhood tumours are relatively more malignant, disseminating early but responding well to therapy in most instances.

Leukaemia

This is nearly always acute lymphoblastic in type. It is commoner in boys and the peak age of onset is from 2 to 5 years. The presentation is likely to result from anaemia causing pallor and lethargy, or from thrombocytopenia causing purpura and bleeding. Fever is common and leukaemic deposits in the bones may cause limb pain. Lymphadenopathy, hepatomegaly and splenomegaly are variable, and frequently not present at onset.

Although the diagnosis must be confirmed by bone marrow examination, it is usually possible to make a presumptive diagnosis from examination of the peripheral blood; anaemia and thrombocytopenia are associated with lymphoblast cells. The total white count is more often normal or decreased than raised at onset. The white cell count is the strongest prognostic factor in acute lymphoblastic leukaemia. Children with $<20 \times 10^9$/l total WBC at diagnosis have a good prognosis; whilst those with $>100 \times 10^9$/l will do less well.

Initial treatment consists of induction of remission with vincristine, asparaginase, daunorubicin and prednisolone combined with supportive therapy in the form of blood or platelet concentrates and antibiotics. 95% of children will achieve a remission within 1 month and be active and happy by then.

Because meningeal leukaemia is a common complication, treatment to induce remission must be followed by intrathecal methotrexate, sometimes with cranial irradiation. Remission is maintained with intermittent cycles of chemotherapy for 2 to 3 years. With modern aggressive therapy, 70% of children are free of disease 5 years after diagnosis; relapse is rare after that time.

Children with acute myeloid leukaemia have a much less favourable outcome. Remission can be achieved in 80% using intensive chemotherapy regimens. For those in remission bone marrow transplantation offers the best chance of cure—60% will then survive compared with 30% survival without transplantation.

Bone marrow transplantation

The child's bone marrow is ablated with high doses of chemotherapy and radiotherapy. Then bone marrow from either a donor (allograft) or from previously stored marrow from the patient (autograft) is infused. Bone marrow allograft from an HLA matched related donor is the treatment of choice for acute myeloid leukamia, poor prognosis lymphoblastic leukaemia, aplastic anaemia, severe combined immunodeficiency and some rare inborn errors of metabolism. Unfortunately only one third of children have a suitably matched sibling donor. When there is no sibling donor an allograft from a matched unrelated donor can be used or, for leukaemia, an autograft.

Lymphomas

These diseases are classified into Hodgkin's disease and non-Hodgkin's lymphoma. Each of these has several histological subdivisions but for treatment purposes only the two major categories need be considered. Hogkin's disease is treated with radiotherapy and/or chemotherapy following careful evaluation of the extent of the disease. The prognosis is good. Non-Hogkin's lymphoma is almost always generalized. It must be treated with intensive multiple drug chemotherapy and has a less good prognosis. Sixty per cent of children will achieve prolonged remission.

Central nervous system tumours

These are most commonly gliomas, either astrocytomas or medulloblastomas. They are mainly situated infratentorially and present with cerebellar signs (ataxia, incoordination, nystagmus) or raised intracranial pressure. In the young child the raised intracranial pressure will cause head enlargement and a bulging fontanelle, whilst in the older child with fused cranial sutures, pain and vomiting will be earlier symptoms. Papilloedema is an important early sign. 'Scanning' by computer-assisted tomography will localize the tumour (younger children may need a general anaesthetic to be sufficiently still for the test).

The treatment is primarily surgical as complete excision of tumour offers the best hope of cure. Radiotherapy and/or chemotherapy may be used to eliminate residual disease, but the prognosis is poor.

Neuroblastoma

This is a malignant tumour arising from the sympathetic nervous tissue. It commonly arises from the adrenal gland but can arise in cervical, thoracic or lumbar sympathetic chains. The tumour presents as an abdominal mass most commonly, but early metastasis (to bone, liver and skin) is the rule, and these may be the presenting signs. An increased output of catecholamine degradation products (e.g. vanillylmandelic acid, HMMA) is usually present in the urine.

Chemotherapy is combined with radiotherapy and surgery. The outlook is poor except for the majority of those who present with localized disease, and also for some children under 1 year of age.

Wilms' tumour (nephroblastoma)

Nephroblastomas are embryonic renal tumours which usually present as a unilateral abdominal mass early in childhood. Microscopic haematuria occurs in up to one third of cases, but macroscopic haematuria is rare. Intravenous urogram shows a distorted kidney. Treatment often achieves complete cure.

Rhabdomyosarcoma

This tumour of striated muscle occurs in many different sites, but commonly is found in the genitourinary tract, the posterior abdominal wall, the nasopharynx or on the extremities. It is treated with a combination of chemotherapy, radiotherapy and surgery. The prognosis is good for tumours of the orbit and genitourinary tract but less good for tumours in the nasopharynx, abdominal wall or limbs.

Bone tumours

Ewing's sarcoma and osteosarcoma usually occur in the long bones and present with pain, swelling or a pathological fracture. Treatment is aimed at surgical excision of the tumour followed by endoprosthetic replacement of the bone and joint, thereby avoiding amputation. The children receive chemotherapy before and after surgery; radiotherapy may be required also. Half the children achieve long-term survival.

TREATMENT OF CHILDHOOD MALIGNANCY

There have been dramatic improvements in treatment and survival over the last 20 years; currently more than 60% of children are cured. As survival increases, the adverse effects of treatment are more apparent. These result more from the medical treatments than from the surgical where there has been an increasing trend away from mutilating surgery. Chemotherapy and radiotherapy are usually combined with surgery and, in the short-term, there may be dangerous immunosuppression and, in the long-term, complications such as pituitary dysfunction, growth failure and neurodevelopmental problems as a result of cranial irradiation, and damage to the heart, kidneys and gonads from chemotherapy. A small proportion develop another primary tumour later in adult life.

Social and psychological problems for the child, their siblings and the family are inevitable. Because of the diversity and complications of treatment childhood malignancy is best treated in a specialized centre where there is a multidisciplinary team available to care for the child and family. This expertise is just as important for the child whose disease cannot be cured, where every effort is made for the child to be cared for at home.

Children's hospices, which may be used for those who cannot be cared for at home, are also used for intermittent respite care, thus providing continued support for the family.

FURTHER READING

Jones PG and Campbell PE. *Tumours of Infancy and Childhood*. Blackwell Scientific Publications.

Chapter 19
Endocrine and Metabolic Disorders

The essential difference between endocrine function in children and in adults is its importance in relation to physical and mental development. The relationships between the various glands, the controlling role of the pituitary, and the feedback mechanisms, are established in prenatal life. This chapter is not intended as a comprehensive catalogue of all the endocrine diseases that can occur in children, but as an indication of those which are most important in childhood or which differ significantly in their presentation or management in children.

HYPOTHYROIDISM

Normal thyroid function is necessary for normal physical and mental growth. Congenital absence of functional thyroid tissue causes *cretinism* which in turn leads to dwarfing and mental deficiency unless promptly recognized and treated. Lesser degrees of hypothyroidism may develop at any time during childhood.

A cretin is not recognizable as such at birth, so all newborns should be screened at birth by measurement of T4 or TSH on a blood spot (in practice this is combined with a screening test for phenylketonuria). In the absence of neonatal screening, suspicions may be aroused by prolonged physiological jaundice or, after a few weeks, lethargy, poor feeding, constipation, umbilical hernia, enlarg-

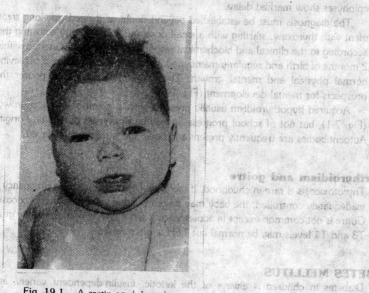

Fig. 19.1. A cretin aged 4 weeks.

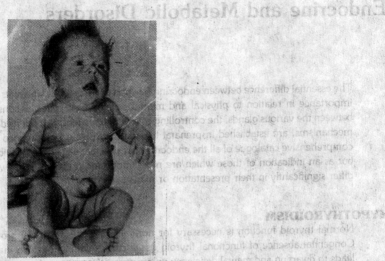

Fig. 19.2.   A cretin aged 4 months. She has coarse features, dry mottled skin, scanty hair and an umbilical hernia.

ing tongue and hoarse cry. Early diagnosis is so important that there should never be the slightest hesitation in investigating a baby on suspicion. The facial appearance is characteristic to the trained eye (Fig. 19.1). Plasma thyroxine (T4) is low, TSH raised (unless the pituitary is at fault) and X-rays of relevant epiphyses show marked delay.

The diagnosis must be established beyond doubt as it needs life-long treatment with thyroxine, starting with a small dose and subsequently adjusting this according to the clinical and biochemical response. If treatment is started within 2 months of birth and regularly maintained, there is a good chance of achieving normal physical and mental growth. The longer the delay, the poorer the prospects for mental development (Fig. 19.2).

Acquired hypothyroidism usually presents with a fall-off of physical growth (Fig. 7.1), but not of school progress. It may be of thyroid or pituitary origin. Autoantibodies are frequently present and bone age is markedly delayed.

Hyperthyroidism and goitre

Thyrotoxicosis is rare in childhood. If maternal hyperthyroidism in pregnancy is inadequately controlled, the baby may be born with self-limiting thyrotoxicosis. Goitre is not common except in adolescence when it affects predominantly girls. T3 and T4 levels may be normal but TSH is often raised.

DIABETES MELLITUS

Diabetes in children is always of the ketotic, insulin-dependent variety, and diabetic children are almost always thin when first diagnosed. They usually present with a short history of polyuria, thirst and weight loss, or in pre-coma.

There may be a family history of diabetes. The diagnosis is confirmed by demonstrating glucose and ketones in the urine and a high blood glucose level. The management of diabetes and coma in children is based on the same principles that apply to adult insulin-dependent diabetes. The following points are particularly relevant to children.

1 Carbohydrate intake must be carefully regulated, but the total calorie intake must be sufficient to maintain normal growth and to allow normal physical activities.

2 The child must learn to manage his own disease as soon as possible.

Children of school age can usually manage to use blood glucose test strips and should do them at least once a day, varying the time at which the test is done and keeping a record of the result to show the supervising doctor. (An index of control over the previous 3 months can be obtained by a periodic estimation of either glycosylated haemoglobin or serum fructosamine.)

There are many different types of insulin, ranging from those with a rapid, brief action to those acting slowly for over 24 hours. Even with mixed short- and long-acting insulins, most diabetic children need insulin twice a day for good control. Some need it more often, and continuous insulin infusion pumps are being developed. Injection technique and regular inspection of injection sites are important. An intelligent 7-year-old can give his own injections under supervision. All diabetic children should experience hypoglycaemia in hospital so that they can recognize it and know what to do about it.

3 The family must be helped to take diabetes in their stride so that it does not interfere with a normal way of life. Membership of the British Diabetic Association is helpful. The Association runs holiday camps for diabetic children. Health visitors specializing in diabetes are a great asset.

4 Diabetes in many children is less stable than in adults. Occasional periods of high blood sugar are almost inevitable if hypoglycaemia is to be avoided. Insulin dosage often has to be reduced after the disease has first been brought under control, and increased at times of infection.

5 Depression is common in diabetic adolescents. The discipline of diabetes is particularly irksome at this age. They may break dietary rules, cheat on tests or omit insulin.

THE ADRENAL GLANDS

Disorders of the adrenal gland are uncommon in children. The least rare is the adrenogenital syndrome. Total adrenocortical insufficiency (Addison's disease) is very rare. Adrenal cortical tumours may secrete androgens or oestrogens, with consequent appearance of the corresponding secondary sexual characteristics. Excess glucocorticoids and mineralocorticoids produce the clinical picture of Cushing's syndrome and may result from administered corticosteroids or (rarely) from adenoma, carcinoma or hyperplasia of the adrenals.

The adrenogenital syndrome

This results from a metabolic block in the synthesis of hydrocortisone, the enzyme defect occuring in individuals homozygous for an autosomal recessive

gene. The fetal adrenal normally secretes hydrocortisone, and the pituitary–
adrenal axis is functional in prenatal life. This disorder therefore has its origins
before birth.

Hydrocortisone deficiency causes increased production of ACTH by the
pituitary. This causes adrenal hyperplasia and excessive production of androgens. The affected female is therefore born with a variable degree of masculinization such as enlarged clitoris and labial fusion. The genitalia of affected boys
look anatomically normal at birth but may be pigmented. Many affected children
lack mineralocorticoids and early in life (often about the 2nd week) develop
symptoms of salt loss—vomiting, dehydration, and collapse. This is lethal if not
recognized and treated. In boys who are not salt-losers, diagnosis is likely to be
delayed until it is recognized that both physical and sexual development are
advancing with excessive speed (infant Hercules). Excessive androgens cause
precocious pseudopuberty, advanced bone growth and advanced epiphyseal
development. In untreated cases, epiphyseal fusion occurs very early and ulti-
mate stature is therefore small.

In cases presenting as intersex, chromosomes show a normal female pattern
and there are raised levels of androgen metabolites and hydrocortisone precursors (17-oxosteroids and 17α-OH progesterone) in blood and urine. Lowered
serum sodium and chloride, with raised potassium levels are found in salt-losers.
Some affected children are hypertensive.

Treatment is essentially the oral replacement of missing hormones. Corticosteroids are required by all patients, with additional fludrocortisone for the
salt-losers. Careful monitoring of dosage is essential and treatment must be
lifelong, with increased dosage at times of stress. Plastic surgery to correct labial
fusion or to recess a large clitoris is carried out in infancy: further surgery at
puberty may be needed.

Cushing's syndrome

This is most commonly seen in children who have been treated with steroids for
long periods (Fig. 19.3). The face is fat and plethoric and there is excess facial
hair. The whole body is obese and there are striae, especially on the abdomen.
There may be hypertension or glycosuria. The effect of endogenous steroids on
growth is variable, but an important hazard of long-term steroid administration is
growth retardation (see p. 227).

Growth hormone deficiency

Deficiency of growth hormone (GH) is an uncommon but important cause of
growth failure. It may be isolated or associated with deficiency of other pituitary
hormones: it may be partial or complete: it is sometimes secondary to an
identifiable intracranial lesion. A useful screening test for GH production involves
a 20-minute period of strenuous exercise, a single blood sample being taken 10
minutes later. Definitive diagnosis requires full endocrine investigation and, if
confirmed, a search for a cause. Genetically engineered human GH is available
for treatment, which needs expert supervision. Growth hormone has also been

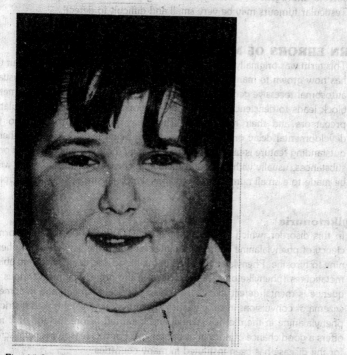

Fig. 19.3. Cushing's syndrome from prolonged corticosteroid therapy. The face is round, hirsute and plethoric.

used to treat short children without demonstrable GH deficiency, with limited success. This also needs expert supervision.

Diabetes insipidus

This is a rare disease resulting from either failure of the hypothalamus to produce sufficient antidiuretic hormone (ADH) or failure of the renal tubule to respond to it (nephrogenic diabetes insipidus). In either case there is marked thirst and the passage of large volumes of almost colourless urine of low osmolality. There is a constant danger of serious water depletion, especially in hot weather, and growth is retarded. ADH deficiency may result from a variety of intracranial disorders, including tumours, cysts, vascular accidents, and meningitis. It may also result from an isolated hormone deficiency, genetically determined. In ADH-deficient cases, desmopressin or pitressin can be given by injection, or intranasally. Nephrogenic diabetes insipidus is caused by an X-linked gene and therefore occurs only in males.

The gonads

Gonadal dysgenesis and testicular feminization are described elsewhere (p. 91), as are undescended testicles (p. 201). Gonadal tumours are very rare. They may secrete androgens or oestrogens, leading to masculinization or feminization. Testicular tumours may be very small and difficult to detect.

INBORN ERRORS OF METABOLISM

This term was originally coined by Garrod to embrace three disorders but the list has now grown to many hundreds. Most are genetically determined, usually by autosomal recessive genes, and most are extremely rare. In some, the metabolic block leads to deficiency of metabolites beyond the block and accumulation of precursors and their metabolites. They may present with failure to thrive, developmental delay or deterioration, fits or acute liver disease. In others, the outstanding feature is failure of reabsorption by the renal tubules of one or more substances, usually with profound metabolic consequences. Reference will only be made to a small number of conditions which illustrate general principles.

Phenylketonuria

In this disorder, which affects about 1 in 10 000–20 000 children born, deficiency of phenylalanine hydroxylase interferes with the conversion of phenylalanine to tyrosine. Phenylalanine levels in the blood and tissues rise, and abnormal metabolites (phenylketones) are excreted in the urine. The most serious consequence is mental defect, but there is also physical stunting, and in some cases eczema or convulsions in early infancy. Treatment by the controlled restriction of phenylalanine in the diet is essential and if started before the age of 2 months offers a good chance of normal development. For this reason neonatal screening for the disease has been instituted in many countries.

Dietetic management is difficult. It aims to maintain serum phenylalanine levels within acceptable limits. Some relaxation of diet can be allowed after 10 years of age, but if a normal diet is resumed too soon behavioural disorders are common. Adult phenylketonuric women may give birth to mentally retarded (though not phenylketonuric) children, presumably because of damage to the fetal brain by high levels of phenylalanine crossing the placenta, and their children are more prone to birth defects (e.g. congenital heart disease). Dietetic restrictions should therefore be resumed before conception and throughout pregnancy.

Galactosaemia

Although some centres screen all infants for galactosaemia, it is not widely practised because of its rarity. Affected babies become ill almost as soon as they begin to drink milk. A deficiency of galactose-1-phosphate uridyl transferase leads to accumulation of galactose in the blood and tissues and its excretion in the urine. Early symptoms are vomiting, weight loss, jaundice and hepatomegaly. Galactose (a reducing sugar) appears in the urine, provided sufficient milk feeds have been taken and retained. Hypoglycaemia may also be evident, and untreated survivors later show mental defect, cataract and cirrhosis of the liver, with hepatoma developing in some. Treatment is by the exclusion of lactose from the diet. The response is good for physical growth, less good for intellectual growth.

RENAL TUBULAR DEFECTS

In this group of disorders, also genetically determined, there is failure of tubular reabsorption of one or more essential substances. Reference is made on p. 219 to nephrogenic diabetes insipidus, which is a defect of tubular reabsorption of water. Phosphate, bicarbonate, glucose and amino acids are lost in other disorders.

Cystinuria

There is tubular loss of cystine and other dibasic amino acids, which may lead to the formation of recurrent urinary calculi. The condition should not be confused with the serious disorder of cystinosis (see below).

Renal tubular acidosis

The classification is complex and is based upon the section of the nephron which is functioning abnormally. However most types present in infancy, or early life, with anorexia, vomiting and failure to thrive as a result of the acidosis. For most types the acidosis can be controlled with alkali supplement.

Fanconi syndrome

This comprises a combination of several tubular defects leading to glycosuria, decreased phosphate reabsorption and hypophosphataemia, amino-aciduria, bicarbonate loss causing acidosis, and potassium and sodium loss. There are many different causes of which the commonest is cystinosis. Cystinosis is subject to autosomal recessive inheritance and is associated with excess cystine storage in the body tissues. In early life there is vomiting and failure to thrive; rickets is common and despite dietary modification and electrolyte supplements the children grow poorly. Renal failure develops in later childhood. Cystine crystals are deposited in the cornea and subsequently cause photophobia; their presence forms a useful diagnostic test on slit-lamp examination.

HYPOGLYCAEMIA

Hypoglycaemia is not a disease but a symptom. The maintenance of normal blood glucose levels depends upon the ingestion, absorption and metabolism of carbohydrates, and normal levels of insulin, glucocorticoids and other hormones. A wide variety of diseases may therefore be associated with hypoglycaemia. Early symptoms include hunger, irritability, pallor, sweating and tachycardia. Later symptoms include convulsions, especially before breakfast, and coma.

Hypoglycaemia in the newborn is most often seen in low birthweight babies (especially the light-for-dates) and in the infants of diabetic mothers (p. 75).

Amongst metabolic disorders, hypoglycaemia is a feature of galactosaemia and some types of glycogen storage disease (a group of genetically determined disorders of glycogen metabolism). It may also occur during the pre-diabetic phase of diabetes mellitus in children. Insulin overdosage is, of course, the commonest cause of hypoglycaemia.

A few infants develop hypoglycaemia after ingestion of leucine, isoleucine or valine. The attacks therefore tend to be post-prandial. Children with hypopituitarism from any cause may have hypoglycaemic episodes and are unduly sensitive to insulin.

Repeated hypoglycaemic fits may lead to brain damage and must therefore be treated vigorously. Emergency treatment consists of the slow intravenous injection of 50% glucose solution, which will rapidly stop fits and restore consciousness. The underlying cause must be sought and if possible treated. If the fundamental cause cannot be treated, diazoxide, steroids or ACTH may be helpful.

FURTHER READING

Brook C. *Clinical Paediatric Endocrinology*. CV Mosby.
Baum JD and Kinmonth AL. *Care of the Child with Diabetes*. Churchill Livingstone.
Hughes IA. *Handbook of Endocrine Tests in Childhood*. Wright.
Sinclair L. *Metabolic Disease in Childhood*. Blackwell Scientific Publications.

Chapter 20
Therapeutics

Therapeutics is not to be regarded as synonymous with the prescription of drugs. Drugs often have an important role, but therapy includes all measures taken to relieve symptoms and to hasten recovery. In the management of medical (as distinct from surgical) conditions in children, the doctor's function is almost entirely advisory, the therapy being carried out largely by the mother at home or by nurses in hospital. Some problems need the help of specialized therapists (e.g. physiotherapists, speech therapists, occupational therapists).

GENERAL MEASURES

In any acute illness advice needs to be given about some basic aspects of management, and a worried mother caring for a sick child at home will appreciate clear guidance.

1 *Rest.* A child who feels ill will want to rest; one who feels well will not. There are very few indications for trying to enforce rest. Active disease of the heart or lungs may restrict activity, as will painful joints, but enforced inactivity will almost alway do more harm than good. At home, the sofa or a comfortable chair downstairs with the TV set is more conducive to rest than bored isolation in the bedroom.

2 *Temperature and humidity.* There is still a lingering fear that febrile children may suffer from chilling, so some parents switch on bedroom heaters and pile on blankets. Such measures can only raise body temperature and increase discomfort and the risk of febrile convulsion in young children. Room temprature should be comfortable (about 18°C, 65°F), preferably with an open window. High fever in a young child is an indication for active cooling by giving antipyretics, removing blankets, using fans and, if necessary, tepid sponging.

Dry air is irritating to an inflamed respiratory tract and may aggravate coughs. Central heating often dries the air and this can be overcome by placing a reservoir of water by the radiator. Cold humidification may give relief in laryngitis. High humidity can only be achieved in a tent. There is no evidence that humidification is helpful in chest infections.

A sheltered corner of a sunny garden is a far better place than a bedroom for convalescence.

3 *Diet.* During acute illnesses, especially febrile illnesses, drinking is more important than eating. The child should be encouraged to drink frequent small quantities of water, fruit juice or glucose drinks. A vomiting child should have a small drink after each vomit: some will return with the next vomit, but some will stay down. Fluid intake may need to be more accurately controlled and recorded in renal disease, and output should be recorded in renal disease and heart failure.

It does not matter if a sick child eats little or nothing for a few days. The lost weight will soon be regained. Appetite is a good guide, and a little of what the child fancies will probably do good. Returning appetite is a good sign of returning health. In some renal disorders, diabetes mellitus, coeliac disease and inborn errors of metabolism, more strictly controlled diets are needed.

4   *Isolation.* Children with infectious diseases nursed at home do not necessarily need to be isolated. Measles and chicken pox are highly infectious before the spots appear, and siblings are probably already infected when the rash develops. With rubella, the risk to pregnant women must be remembered.

5   *Schoolwork.* To miss any substantial time from school may set back a child's educational progress, especially if this happens around the time of crucial examinations. In most hospitals teachers are made available by education authorities to work on children's wards. At home, teachers are usually glad to provide schoolwork and will sometimes call in to help with problems. For children confined to their homes for long periods (a rare event today), the education authority can provide a home teacher. Children who have been ill should be allowed back to school as soon as possible, if necessary on a part-time basis initially, but physical activities (games and PE) may need to be postponed for longer.

DRUGS

When these general points have been attended to, more often than not it will be appropriate to prescribe one or more drugs. In spite of the enormous number of drugs and compounds available, the wise doctor will confine his prescribing to a relatively small number of drugs with which he is familiar. The newest drug is not necessarily the best, and is certainly the one of which there is least experience. An old remedy is not necessarily a bad one. Experienced doctors find that they can treat all but the most obscure conditions with fewer than fifty drugs.

In the UK, accurate up-to-date information and advice on prescribing is most readily found in the British National Formulary (BNF) which is distributed to all doctors free of charge.

The prescription of a drug for a patient is often done with little thought at all, but if medicine is to be practised at its best, it demands a 10-point catechism.

1   *Is a drug necessary?* Am I treating a symptom or the underlying disease, or am I prescribing a placebo to make anxious parents or myself feel better? Is this a virus infection? (because if so antibiotics are unnecessary).

2   *If so, which one?* If an antibiotic, what organisms are likely to be involved and what will be effective against them? What drug has the best chance of doing good without doing harm? Prefer a familiar drug to an unfamiliar. Other things being equal, economize. The use of generic names may save money.

3   *Which preparation shall I use?* Try to find something palatable for young children. Do not order capsules for babies unless it is permissible to put the contents in a spoon. Some young children prefer tablets; some older ones prefer medicines. Ask the mother. Avoid using sucrose-based syrups long-term—they rot teeth.

4   *What route of administration?* Do not give injections if they can be avoided, but they may be necessary if the child is vomiting or if it is necessary to achieve high tissue levels quickly. If there is peripheral circulatory failure, drugs given by intramuscular injection may be absorbed slowly. If there is serious infection

(meningitis, septicaemia), give antibiotics intravenously to begin with.

5   *How much, how often, for how long?* There is no infallible formula for calculating dosage for children. The younger the child, the more critical the dose (especially the newborn baby). There is a big margin of safety for some drugs, but very little for others, such as digoxin. Therefore, put the child's age or date of birth on the prescription. This gives the pharmacist a chance to check the dose. Frequency of administration depends on the duration of action of the drug. Do not disturb sleep unnecessarily. Arrange an infant's drug schedule to fit in with the feeding schedule (i.e. avoid ordering 6-hourly drugs and 4-hourly feeds). Remember to specify the duration of treatment.

6   *Is the drug compatible with the patient?* Is there any history of drug allergy or other untoward reaction? Has he any disorder that limits the use of any drugs (e.g. glucose-6-phosphate dehydrogenase deficiency)?

7   *Is the drug compatible with other durgs?* If two or more drugs are being given, ensure that they do not inhibit or potentiate one another. Be especially careful of mixing drugs for intravenous administration.

8   *Have I written the prescription legibly?*

9   *Have I given any necessary instructions about the administration of the drug or its storage (preferably in writing)?*

10   *Have I given any necessary warning of side-effects*, whether harmless (e.g. dark stools with iron) or serious?

A general indication of the drugs appropriate for the treatment of common conditions will be found in the other chapters of this book, but some comments on common prescribing problems are included here. In most clinical situations there is no one line of treatment that is undoubtedly superior to all others and you may therefore meet a bewildering variety of therapeutic approaches amongst your medical teachers. Sometimes you may meet direct conflict, one teacher advising you never to do something that another habitually does. Have courage and ask the reason why.

Prescribing for the newborn

Very few drugs are needed for the treatment of neonatal disease, and some are positively harmful. Many of the metabolic functions of the liver and the excretory capacity of the kidneys take a week or so to develop fully. During this time very high blood levels of drugs may be achieved on relatively low dosage. This is especially true of the preterm infant. Sulphonamides and tetracyclines should be avoided altogether. Serious infections at this age are usually caused by Gram-negative bacteria and group B streptococci and are best treated with gentamicin combined with ampicillin or penicillin. Naloxone (0.2 mg i.m.) is an antidote to morphine and pethidine. Irritability and convulsions due to cerebral problems may be controlled with phenobarbitone but if due to metabolic disturbances (e.g. hypoglycaemia) appropriate correction must be made.

Oxygen is a powerful therapeutic weapon. In the severely asphyxiated newborn, endotracheal oxygen is the most pressing need. In respiratory and some cardiac problems, the intelligent use of oxygen is crucial. But excessive concentrations of oxygen can damage the eyes and the lungs. Monitoring of blood gases is therefore essential.

Iron and vitamin supplements are needed by all preterm babies. It is not *necessary* to start them before 6 weeks, and little iron is absorbed before this time, but it is *convenient* to start them before the baby is discharged home.

Remember that drugs given to pregnant women are being given to unborn babies. Though most drugs given to a mother are excreted, to some extent, in her breast milk it is unusual for them to affect the baby.

Antibiotics

If there are infections in paradise, the causative organism will be known every time and there will be available an antibiotics which kills that organism and no others. In this life we must make an intelligent guess at the organism (until the laboratory can give us help) and decided what chemotherapy is appropriate. If the infection is certainly or probably viral (measles, influenza, laryngitis), antibiotics are not needed. The notion of 'preventing secondary bacterial infection' is not valid. In some bacterial infections, especially bacillary dysentery, there is good evidence that antibiotics do harm. There may be genuine diagnostic uncertainties, as between bronchiolitis (viral) and bronchopneumonia (viral or bacterial) in infants.

If swabs or samples of urine, faeces, blood or CSF are needed for culture, take them before starting antibiotics. Swabs, unless of frank pus, need to be taken thoroughly, transported expeditiously and incubated promptly.

Some antibiotics cause diarrhoea, others (especially ampicillin) cause rashes. Such symptoms often settle in spite of continuation of the drug. Babies given broad-spectrum antibiotics often develop oral thrush (moniliasis). Tetracyclines should be avoided under the age of 12 years because they damage and discolour the teeth.

If an unnecessary antibiotic has been started, stop it as soon as possible.

Anticonvulsants

Children metabolize anticonvulsant drugs faster than adults so that a single daily dose is less likely to be effective in childhood. An additional problem with phenobarbitone is that it causes hyperkinesis and behavioural problems in some children. Both phenytoin and phenobarbitone predispose to rickets, particularly in institutionalized children receiving a poor diet and little sunshine.

Plasma drug levels give an indication of the adequacy of the dose but can only be interpreted if the time between last dose and blood sampling is known. Undetectable levels suggest noncompliance.

Sodium valproate, ethosuximide and carbamazepine are *relatively* free from side-effects. Phenytoin nearly always causes some gum hyperplasia which goes when the drug is stopped. Children taking it need good dental care. Hirsutism and ataxia are not uncommon. More subtle, but important, side-effects to watch for and enquire about include impaired school performance, personality change and disturbed behaviour.

Sedatives and tranquillizers

It should only exceptionally be necessary to prescribe these drugs for children. Tranquillizers are sometimes needed for children with behavioural disorders, but they should only be used as an adjunct to attempts to determine and influence the cause of the misbehaviour.

Steroids

Cortisone and its many relatives may be used either locally or systemically, for short- or long-term treatment. Local steroids include many preparations for the treatment of skin conditions (e.g. hydrocortisone for eczema), for inhalation (e.g. beclamethasone for asthma), and in eye drops. The quantities of steroid absorbed from these preparations appears to be minimal, except when used for extensive eczema.

Short-term oral or parenteral steroids are valuable in the treatment of severe asthmatic attacks, overwhelming infections and allergic reactions. In these critical situations, large doses should be given, but can soon be stopped.

Medium-term (weeks or months) oral steroids are used to induce remissions in leukaemia, the nephrotic syndrome and some autoimmune disorders. During treatment, excessive weight gain, plethora and hirsutism commonly develop, but subside when treatment is stopped. More serious side-effects are rare.

Long-term (years) oral steroids are rarely needed. Stunting of height may be reduced by giving intermittent (e.g. alternate day) steroids. Single daily doses are best given in the morning to fit in with the normal circadian rhythm. Excessive weight gain can be prevented by calorie control, but this is difficult to achieve.

After medium- and long-term therapy, steroid dosage should be reduced gradually. The normal pituitary response to stress may be impaired for some months thereafter, so steroid cover for operations, etc. is needed.

Salicylates

Aspirin is no longer recommended as an analgesic and antipyretic for children under 12 years of age because of a possible link with Reye's syndrome (p. 174). Paracetamol or ibuprofen should be used instead.

In rheumatic fever salicylates have a specific effect, but should be given in maximal dosage for maximal relief (see p. 182). They are also used for rheumatoid arthritis (p. 180) and here again large doses may be necessary.

FURTHER READING

Gellis SS and Kagan BM. *Current Pediatric Therapy.* WB Saunders.
Insley J. *A Paediatric Vade-Mecum.* Lloyd-Luke.
Maxwell GM *Principles of Paediatric Pharmacology.* Oxford University Press.
Shirkey HC. *Pediatric Therapy.* CV Mosby.

Chapter 21
Immunity, Immunization and Specific Fevers

Most illness in childhood is infective, and an important activity in the early life of every individual is meeting and establishing immunity to a wide variety of infecting organisms. Immunological mechanisms in childhood are essentially the same as in adults but are not fully developed at birth. Cellular immunity is effective from birth: for the first 2 or 3 years of life, lymphocytes predominate over polymorphs in the circulating blood, but the total white cell count is relatively high (p. 204). Pus can be formed at any age. Humoral immunity is slower to develop. Maternal IgG is transferred across the placenta from early fetal life, and in the full-term infant approximates to adult levels. This conveys passive immunity to a number of common infections, including measles, rubella and mumps. In contrast, the larger molecules of IgM do not cross the placenta and the neonate is therefore fully susceptible to bacterial infections including pertussis. The fetus is capable of making its own IgM in response to intrauterine infection, e.g. rubella, but synthesis of other immunoglobulins gets off to a rather sluggish start after birth. A reasonable level of humoral immunity is established by the age of 6–9 months (Fig. 21.1).

Preterm babies have relatively low levels of circulating immunoglobulins and are particularly susceptible to infection but they can mount a satisfactory response to vaccines. Total immunoglobulin levels in all infants reach their lowest at about 3–4 months of age which is another susceptible period. In older

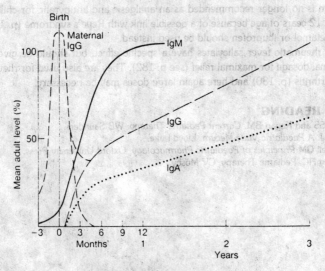

Fig. 21.1. Immunoglobulin levels in early life.

children, recurrent infections are rarely due to immunological deficiencies. Poor social conditions and debilitating diseases such as cystic fibrosis or congenital heart disease may predispose to infection. Recurrent skin infections may be associated with nasal carriage of *Staphylococcus pyogenes*, and recurrent urinary infections with congenital anomalies of the renal tract. Rarely, however, repeated infections, especially of the skin and lungs, may be due to some defect of the cellular or humoral defence mechanisms.

IMMUNIZATION

In the UK, authoritative information and advice about all aspects of immunization are to be found in the HMSO publication 'Immunization against Infectious Disease' ('the green book') which is available to all doctors free of charge. It is updated regularly.

As infectious diseases account for a large part of the mortality and morbidity of early childhood, it is imperative to make the maximum use of all available preventive measures. All doctors responsible for children must impress on parents the necessity for full immunization, and must themselves be committed to pursuing such a policy with enthusiasm. Britain has a poor track record in the immunization field, although it is currently improving. This has been as much due to health personnel observing fictitious contraindications as to parental misgivings.

Table 21.1 shows the programme of immunization currently recommended for children in the UK. In determining such a schedule, two basic decisions need to be made.

1   Against what diseases should a child be protected? This requires a balance of the probabilities of him catching it, suffering death or disability from it and the dangers and effectiveness of the immunizing procedure. The more common and the more dangerous the disease, and the safer the immunization, the greater the need.

Table 21.1. Programme of immunization currently recommended in the UK.

Vaccine	Age	Notes
Diphtheria/tetanus/pertussis (DTP) and polio	1st dose 2 months 2nd dose 3 months 3rd dose 4 months	Primary course
Measles/mumps/rubella (MMR)	12–18 months	Can be given at any age over 12 months
Booster D/T and polio	4–5 years	If not given earlier
Measles/mumps/rubella (MMR)	4–5 years	
Rubella	10–14 years	Girls only
BCG	10–14 years or infancy	Interval of 3 weeks between BCG and rubella
Booster tetanus and polio	15–18 years	

2   At what age should immunization be done? This depends upon the age of susceptibility of the child and the age at which he can best respond to the vaccine. There is often a conflict here, as in the case of pertussis. The greatest danger of the disease is in the first 6 months of life, but the immunological response is relatively poor before 3 months of age. Immunizing procedures should be avoided in children who are unwell, and live vaccine should not be given to those who are immunologically depressed (from disease or drugs). Live vaccine viruses may be transmitted from person to person in a household; the possible risk to pregnant women must be remembered.

Diphtheria

This has become an extremely rare disease in Britain, whereas at the turn of the century it was a major cause of death in childhood. The continuance of this happy state depends upon continuing immunization of all infants. The toxoid scarcely ever causes any disturbance and there are no contraindications to its use in young children. It is normally combined with tetanus and pertussis vaccines (DTP).

Tetanus

Tetanus is rare, but it is still a serious illness and routine immunization is wise. Tetanus toxoid is safe and effective. For primary immunization it is normally combined with diphtheria and pertussis vaccines (DTP).

Pertussis

Pertussis vaccine, prepared from killed whooping cough bacilli, is the third component of triple vaccine and is the only one of the three likely to cause any disturbance of health. Minor reactions are common—restlessness, fever or transient screaming episodes coming on a few hours after the injection. The possibility that pertussis vaccine may cause brain damage very rarely is not resolved but the risk after whooping cough is likely to be greater. Expert advice should be sought before it is given to infants with evidence of disordered brain function (e.g. fits or cerebral palsy).

D/T/P vaccine and its components are given by i.m. or deep subcutaneous injection.

Poliomyelitis

Poliomyelitis vaccine is usually given in the oral form (Sabin vaccine) which contains live virus. Side-effects are practically unknown. The only contraindications are those for live vaccines and *extreme* sensitivity of penicillin, streptomycin, neomycin or polymyxin. It is highly effective.

Measles

Measles vaccination with a live attenuated vaccine is generally safe and effective. A mild measles-like illness may occur after the immunization. Encephalitis is a very rare complication. It is about 10 times more common after natural measles. *Extreme* hypersensitivity to egg protein, neomycin or polymyxin are contraindications.

It is usually given combined with mumps and rubella vaccines (MMR).

Mumps

Mumps vaccine contains live virus and is normally given combined with measles and rubella vaccines (MMR).

Rubella

This is not a danger except to the embryo. In Britain, in addition to MMR vaccination of both sexes at 12–18 months, rubella vaccination is recommended for girls aged 10–14 years, and adult females and selected males who are shown to be non-immune. Immunity usually lasts at least 20 years.

Measles, mumps and rubella vaccines are given by i.m. or deep subcutaneous injection.

BCG

BCG is a live vaccine which gives substantial protection against tuberculosis. It is injected *intradermally* over the insertion of the deltoid muscle. Meticulous technique reduces the risks of infections and keloid scarring. After 3–6 weeks there is local erythema, induration and sometimes ulceration. The axillary glands may enlarge and be painful. The local signs go in 2–6 months. The use of BCG varies greatly in different countries; in some, BCG is given routinely to all infants. In Britain, schoolchildren have a tuberculin test at the age of 10–14 years and those who are tuberculin negative are given BCG. Babies are given BCG during the neonatal period if anyone in the immediate family has had TB.

DIAGNOSIS OF INFECTIONS

In children with unexplained fever and in some in whom a firm 'disease diagnosis' has been made (e.g. meningitis), it is important to try to establish the responsible organism. This may be achieved by the following.

1 Identification of the organism:
  (a) by microscopy;
  (b) by culture.
2 Demonstration of a rise of specific antibody titre.

Direct light microscopy of unstained material from body fluids (e.g. urine, CSF), pus and biopsy specimens, may reveal identifiable bacteria.

Immunofluorescent techniques allow rapid, positive identification. Swabs should be taken thoroughly (especially throat swabs) and transported to the laboratory swiftly. Skin scrapings are needed to identify skin fungi. Blood cultures are best taken when fever is rising. Take all necessary bacteriological specimens before giving antibiotics, if possible. Material for virological culture must be put straight into transport medium.

Demonstration of a significant *rise* in antibody titre, whether bacterial (e.g. ASO) or viral, requires at least two specimens, one taken early in the illness, another 10 days to 3 weeks later. A single convalescent sample showing a high antibody titre must be interpreted more cautiously.

SPECIFIC FEVERS

The main clinical features of the common infectious diseases of childhood together with their incubation periods and important complications are listed in

Table 21.2. Common infectious diseases.

Disease	Incubation period (days)*	Main features	Important complications	Laboratory findings
Measles	7–10–12	Misery, fever, catarrh, cough, conjunctivitis; Koplik's spots, blotchy, red rash on face and trunk	Pneumonia Otitis media Encephalitis	Rise in antibody titre
Rubella	10–18–21	Upper respiratory catarrh; macular or erythematous rash; chiefly on trunk; cervical adenopathy	Virtually none in childhood Encephalitis very rare	Virus culture from stool or nose Rise in antibody titre
Chicken pox	10–14–21	Rash on trunk, perineum and scalp; papules, vesicles, pustules, scabs; fever at pustular stage	Conjunctival lesions Encephalitis	
Mumps	14–18–28	Parotitis, sometimes involvement of other salivary glands	Meningitis Pancreatitis Orchitis after puberty	Virus from saliva Rise in antibody titre Lymphocytosis
Whooping cough	7–10–14	Upper respiratory catarrh; paroxysmal cough with vomiting. Modified greatly by immunization	Pneumonia Lobar collapse Convulsions Haemorrhage (nose, eyes, brain)	B. pertussis from per-nasal swab Lymphocytosis + +
Scarlet fever	1–3–7	Tonsillitis (pharyngitis); diffuse, erythematous rash chiefly on trunk; sore, coated tongue; circumoral pallor	Otitis media Rheumatic fever Acute nephritis	Group A haem. strep. from throat Rise in ASO titre

* Outer figures = range, centred italic figure = usual.

Table 21.2. Infectivity is usually maximal in the prodromal stage and ends within a week of definitive signs appearing. The following paragraphs describe the aspects of these diseases which are important in childhood.

Measles (morbilli)

This usually presents with respiratory catarrh, misery, fever and a red, maculo-papular rash which starts behind the ears; less frequent presentations include febrile convulsion and epistaxis. Sometimes the prodrome appears prolonged, with unexplained, intermittent fever. A prodromal rash, quite unlike a measles rash, may appear at about the time of appearance of Koplik's spots, which are small (pinhead) whitish spots on the mucosa inside the cheeks and lower lip. Otitis media and bronchopneumonia are common complications; encephalitis is rare but serious. In the absence of complications, antibiotics are not indicated.

Rubella (German measles)

Rubella may present with rash, respiratory catarrh, or epistaxis. In general, the illness is very mild and there are virtually no complications. The rash, mainly on the trunk, usually consists of small, pink macules but may be confluent and resemble scarlet fever. The suboccipital lymph glands are usually enlarged. The arthralgia of the hands so common in adolescent and adult females does not affect children.

Chicken pox (varicella)

This is usually a mild disease. The differential diagnosis is from papular urticaria (p. 188) which, if scratched and infected, also presents papules, vesicles, pustules and scabs. However, the lesions in chicken pox are predominantly on the trunk, whilst papular urticaria is peripherally distributed. Complications are rare. Chicken pox encephalitis presents as ataxia a week or so after the rash has appeared; the prognosis is good.

Mumps

This is most commonly confused with cervical adenitis. The exact location of the swelling, the fact that it is nearly always bilateral, the swelling of the orifice of the parotid ducts, and absence of any cause for cervical adenitis, should make the diagnosis clear. Mumps is the commonest cause of lymphocytic meningitis, and can occur without parotitis. Rarely nerve deafness occurs, usually unilateral. Pancreatitis and orchitis are rare before puberty.

Whooping cough (pertussis)

Whooping cough is a serious disease in the very young infant, and unpleasant at all ages. Babies with pertussis do not whoop, but the cough is paroxysmal and associated with vomiting. Infants may present with an apnoea attack, a day or two before the cough develops. Severe spasms may lead to capillary rupture (which is common in the conjunctivae) or may lead to hypoxia sufficient to cause a convulsion. Lobar collapse is not uncommon.

Encephalopathy is rare. In children who have been immunized, the disease tends to be mild, the whoop absent, and there may be no lymphocytosis; the diagnosis is then easily missed

Scarlet fever (scarlatina)

This has become a rare disease since the introduction of penicillin. See Table 21.2.

Roseola infantum (exanthem subitum)

Roseola infantum is a mild disease of infants and young children, common outside hospital but rarely severe enough to need admission. Catarrhal symptoms and fever for 3 or 4 days are followed by the abrupt appearance of light red, discrete macules on the trunk. As the rash appears, the fever rapidly settles and the child is greatly improved. A few days later, the illness is over.

Erythema infectiosum (Fifth disease)

This mildly contagious disease is caused by a human parvovirus. It commences on the face with bright red cheeks ('slapped face'). Subsequently maculopapular red spots appear on the limbs with a symmetrical distribution beginning on the extensor surfaces and spreading to the flexor surfaces and then to the buttocks and trunk. The rash subsides over the course of a week but may recur in response to a variety of skin irritants. Aplastic crises are an important complication in persons who have a chronic haemolytic anaemia.

Infectious mononucleosis (glandular fever)

Glandular fever results from infection with Epstein–Barr virus, but a similar clinical picture may result from infection by several viruses or by *Toxoplasma gondii*.

The presentation is variable: the onset may be gradual with malaise, anorexia and low grade fever for one to two weeks, or it may begin abruptly with high fever and headache. Specific signs include:

1 Lymphadenopathy—multiple, firm, discrete, non-tender glands especially in the neck. They never suppurate.
2 Splenomegaly.
3 Pharyngitis.
4 Rash in some cases, macular or urticarial. Ampicillin often causes a morbilliform rash if given to somebody with glandular fever.
5 Jaundice—resulting from an associated hepatitis or from enlarged glands in the porta hepatis.
6 Meningeal involvement, with headache, stiff neck, and raised cells and protein in the CSF.
7 Haematuria, resulting from a mild glomerulonephritis.

In classic glandular fever, the blood shows an increased number of mononuclear cells (lymphocytes and monocytes) with atypical lymphocytes ('glandular fever cells'). There may be thrombocytopenia. The Paul–Bunnell (heterophil antibody) test is positive after the first week or two of illness. In practice, a simplified version of this test (Monospot) is generally used.

Hepatitis A (infectious hepatitis)

World-wide, this is the commonest cause of jaundice in children over the age of 3 years. It is seen most frequently where hygiene is poor. It tends to be milder in children than in adults. There is a prodromal period lasting about a week, in which malaise, anorexia, abdominal pain and nausea predominate, before jaundice appears. The liver is tender and a little enlarged. The stools are pale, the urine dark, and urine testing reveals the presence of urobilinogen and bile pigment. Urobilinogen may be detected in the pre-icteric stage and may be the sole diagnostic clue in the mildest cases in which clinical jaundice does not develop. Serum bilirubin levels are raised, with roughly equal parts conjugated and free, as are transaminase levels.

Differential diagnosis in the pre-icteric and non-icteric cases is from other causes of abdominal pain and vomiting. Once jaundice has developed, diagnosis is not difficult. Complications are rare. Jaundice usually fades in 1-2 weeks but exceptionally persists for months.

Cross-infection should be prevented as far as possibly by care in handling stools and by conscientious hand-washing by the patient and attendants. However, infectivity is greatest before jaundice appears and it is quite common to have more than one case in a household.

In the average case the child will be in bed for a week and kept off school for 2-3 weeks.

TUBERCULOSIS

Tuberculosis is common wherever poverty, malnutrition and overcrowding are prevalent, and rare where standards of hygiene and nutrition are good. In the developing countries of the world, tuberculosis appears in forms that were common in Britain 50 years ago. The chief sources of infection are adults with sputum-positive pulmonary tuberculosis, and milk from infected cattle. Prevention depends first upon general improvement in socioeconomic conditions, and second upon specific measures including the prompt recognition and treatment of infectious adults, BCG immunization, tuberculin testing of cattle and pasteurization of milk.

The initial infection is in the lungs if conveyed by droplets, in the bowel if conveyed by milk. The first site of infection is known as the primary *focus;* the primary *complex* comprises the primary focus and the enlarged lymph nodes draining it. Spread of infection beyond the local nodes may result in tubercle bacilli reaching the blood stream, causing either tuberculous septicaemia (miliary TB) or infection of distant organs (meninges, kidneys, bones and joints). Tuberculous cervical lymph nodes are thought to be infected via the tonsils. Erythema nodosum may be caused by tuberculosis (p. 188).

In Britain, childhood tuberculosis is uncommon. Primary complexes in the lung are seen more often in immigrant children from Asia than in others, and tuberculous meningitis is a rare disease.

Pulmonary tuberculosis

The child with a primary complex has minimal symptoms. Haemoptysis and systemic symptoms are exceptional. Children with TB, traced through their contact with infected adults, are often completely symptom-free. Diagnosis is based on the X-ray appearances and a positive tuberculin test. Sputum is not usually present, but tubercle bacilli may be recovered from gastric washings.

Tuberculous meningitis

This disease which was universally fatal before the discovery of streptomycin is still a serious disease, especially in infancy. It most commonly affects young children; the onset is insidious so that there is usually a history of weight loss or poor weight gain, initially vague malaise, anorexia and perhaps slight fever. After a few days, evidence of meningeal involvement is shown by headache, drowsiness, irritability and neck stiffness. If the diagnosis is not made at this stage, convulsions, pareses and impairment of consciousness supervene. The clinical signs are those of meningitis (p. 110). In addition, choroidal tubercles may be visible as small yellow lesions close to retinal arteries at the periphery of the retina. The CSF may be hazy, and a cobweb clot forms if the fluid is left undisturbed for 24 hours. The cells are predominantly lymphocytes, but polymorphs may predominate in the early stages. Protein is raised and glucose low. Tubercle bacilli may be seen on suitably stained films of CSF, but their absence does not exclude the diagnosis. A chest X-ray may show a localized lesion or miliary lesions. In very sick children, the tuberculin test may be negative, and this should never be allowed to exclude the diagnosis.

Cervical adenopathy

Tuberculous neck glands are rare in Britain. Usually a single gland or group of glands is affected, on one side of the neck. The gland is firm (unless caseating), partially fixed and not especially tender. The tuberculin test is positive. The differential diagnosis is from Hodgkin's disease, and infection by anonymous mycobacteria, a group of organisms related to the tubercle bacillus but less virulent. Enlarged glands associated with recurrent tonsillitis are usually bilateral, fairly soft and mobile, though occasionally they form a localized abscess requiring drainage.

Management

Regardless of the site, the management of tuberculosis can be divided into three parts.

1   Notification of the case to the local public health specialist so that contacts can be immunized and possible sources of infection identified.
2   Anti-tuberculous drugs. Rifampicin, ethambutol and isoniazid form the basis of treatment in most cases. Treatment should be continued for at least 9 months.
3   General management. Children should not be admitted to hospital or kept off school without good reason. A pulmonary primary complex is rarely infectious, and isolation is unnecessary. If nutrition is unsatisfactory, it should be improved.

MALARIA

Malaria is endemic in many parts of the world (Fig. 21.2) and may be seen in immigrants from malarious areas or in persons who have visited such places but failed to take adequate suppressive drugs. It usually presents with fever which does not necessarily show the classic periodic pattern. The spleen may be enlarged. Diagnosis depends on identification of parasites in blood smears, and may be easier *between* peaks of fever. It may be necessary to examine several smears.

Plasmodium can develop resistance to drugs. The appropriate treatment varies according to the local sensitivity of the responsible organism. Prophylactic drugs must be taken throughout residence in a malarial area *and for at least 4 weeks thereafter.*

NOTIFICATION OF INFECTIOUS DISEASES

Doctors are required, for public health and epidemiological reasons, to notify to the District Medical Officer for Environmental Health a number of infectious diseases, including:

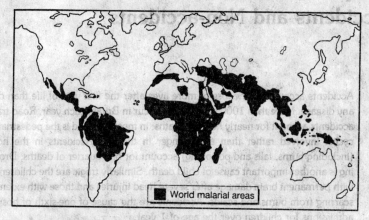

World malarial areas

Fig. 21.2. Distribution of malarial endemic areas.

Diphtheria	Paratyphoid
Dysentery	Poliomyelitis
Encephalitis	Rubella
Food poisoning	Scarlet fever
Hepatitis A and B	Tetanus
Measles	Tuberculosis
Malaria	Typhoid
Meningitis	Varicella/zoster (in Scotland)
Meningococcal infection	Whooping cough
Mumps	

In spite of the payment of a modest fee for each notification, only a small proportion of the more common notifiable diseases are notified. More reliable information is obtained from 'spotter practices' which notify voluntarily to the Royal College of General Practitioners.

FURTHER READING

Department of Health. *Immunisation against Infectious Disease.* HMSO.
Krugman S, Katzsh SL, Gershon AA and Wilfert C. *Infectious Diseases of Children.* CV Mosby.
Marks MI. *Pediatric Infectious Diseases for the Practitioner.* Springer-Verlag.

Chapter 22
Accidents and Non-accidents

Accidents account for the loss of more lives after the first year of life than does any disease. More than 1000 such deaths occur in Britain each year. Road traffic accidents account for nearly half the deaths; in most the child is the pedestrian or cyclist involved rather than a passenger in the car. Accidents in the home (including burns, falls and poisoning) account for one-quarter of deaths. Drowning is another important cause of child death. Similarly tragic are the children left with permanent brain damage after severe head injuries and those with extensive scarring from burns and scalds. Accidents are the cause of one-sixth of hospital admissions for children over the age of 1 year.

Accidents are more common amongst boys than girls. By the age of 11, 1 in 4 children has experienced a serious accident. The risk of accident is influenced by social circumstances. The child in a large family in an industrial slum, on the street much of the day and ostensibly supervised by another child only marginally older, is at great hazard; and the mother trying to care for young children at the top of a tower block, without the privilege of an enclosed garden or play space, has a difficult task. The greatest reduction in mortality and morbidity from accidents will only come about by improved design of towns and homes. Nevertheless, there are many practical things that can be done even in difficult conditions. Pedestrian accidents are commonest in the 5–9 age group when parents are falsely confident about their child's skills: it is wiser to under-, rather than over-, estimate a child's abilities. In general, children cannot cross a busy road safely on their own until the age of 8 or 9 years, and cannot ride a bicycle safely on a main road until 13. Injuries to child passengers in car accidents are reduced by ensuring that infants are transported in carry cots strapped to the back seat and that older children use safety seats or wear a seat belt. (Any child travelling in a car not fitted with a special child restraint and not large enough to wear an adult belt correctly should be placed in the rear seat with the doors locked to reduce the risk of ejection. On no account should children stand on the car seat because of the risk of being thrown violently forward in an accident.)

Fireguards, stairgates and locked medicine cupboards are measures that any wise parent should use. Child-resistant containers for dangerous drugs, and clothes of non-flammable material similarly prevent many accidents. There is great need for better education of children and parents about safety, and for legislation to minimize the opportunities for accidents. Many people feel that it is wrong to enforce the use of protective measures such as seat belts. They feel that individuals should have freedom of choice (regardless of the cost to society or the consequence to others). Children do not have freedom of choice: they cannot choose parents who will be wise, keeping them in a safe environment. Therefore, legislation is required to minimize the opportunities for accidents to children.

HEAD INJURY

The management of head injuries calls for some experience. On the one hand, scalps split easily and bleed profusely, but the quantity of blood may cause unjustifiable alarm. On the other hand, some apparently trivial injuries are associated with intracranial bleeding that only becomes apparent after an interval of time. A history of unconsciousness, however brief, should be regarded seriously. Pallor, vomiting and sleepiness can occur after quite minor injuries, but should settle within an hour or two. Progressive symptoms or the appearance of abnormal neurological signs suggest intracranial injury.

Skull X-rays are often taken, but a linear fracture without displacement may be unimportant, whilst intracranial bleeding may occur without a fracture. In any case of doubt, it is wiser to admit a child with a head injury to hospital for 24 hours' observation, which will include frequent recording of pulse and respiratory rates, blood pressure, level of consciousness and pupillary size and reactions. If there is any suggestion of intracranial bleeding, the opinion of a neurosurgeon should be sought without delay.

BURNS AND SCALDS

Scalds are caused by hot fluids and cause predominantly loss of the epidermis only, with blistering and peeling. However, the skin of young children sometimes suffers full thickness loss from comparatively minor scalds. For this reason there is a strong argument for limiting the maximum temperature of hot water in the home to 52°C (125°F). Most scalds occur in the kitchen; parents should be advised to use electric kettles with short coiled flexes which reduce the risk of a child reaching up and pulling the kettle over.

Burns are caused by direct contact with very hot objects or by the clothes catching fire and result in full thickness skin loss. Burns are the second commonest cause of accidental death in children (after road traffic accidents). The death rate varies with the proportion of the total body surface involved. Loss of skin surface leads to loss of fluid and shock. If more than 10% of the body surface is involved (Fig. 22.1), intravenous fluid therapy will be required. Burns involving 50% or more of the body surface carry a grave prognosis, although children have survived more extensive burns than this.

As a general rule, burns and scalds are more serious than they seem, and hospital admission is advisable for all but the most trivial.

POISONING

The accidental swallowing of drugs and household fluids by young children is extremely common, but few of them become ill and mortality is very low. The majority are 2- and 3-year-olds who are sufficiently agile to get hold of things to swallow, but not old enough to appreciate the dangers. Occasionally younger children are fed with poisons by their siblings or parents. If older children in the prepubertal–adolescent age range swallow poisonous substances (usually drugs), this is indicative of an emotional upset. Most often it is done as a gesture of defiance, or a wish for temporary oblivion, rather than with serious intention to commit suicide. Nevertheless, some are pathologically depressed and the advice of a child psychiatrist should be sought when schoolchildren have swallowed poison.

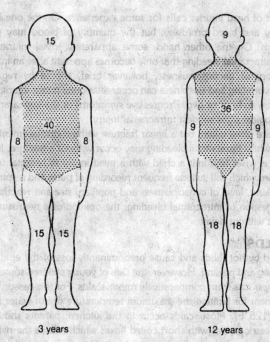

Fig. 22.1. Skin surface areas at 3 and 12 years. The figures indicate the percentage of total body surface represented by each part.

The things that children swallow are numberless, but fall into three main categories:

1 Tablets and medicines: analgesics, sleeping tablets, tranquillizers, antidepressants and iron are commonly ingested. They are a more common cause of morbidity (and mortality) than substances in the other two groups below.

2 Household and horticultural fluids: bleach, turpentine, paraffin, cleaning fluids and weedkillers.

3 Berries and seeds. Laburnum tops the list with deadly nightshade and toadstools featuring commonly. In Britain, things plucked from the hedgerows and ditches hardly ever cause serious illness.

The basis of treatment of poisoning is to minimize absorption, to promote excretion and to combat symptoms. With some important exceptions, the stomach should be emptied by the most efficient means available unless more than 6 hours have elapsed since the poison was swallowed, or unless it is certain that the amount the child may have swallowed could not cause trouble. Most authorities favour induced emesis rather than gastric lavage. It is more effective in removing solid matter (e.g. whole tablets), it is less unpleasant for the child and it occupies less nursing time. Emesis usually follows the administration of 20 ml ipecacuanha syrup in orange juice, repeated if necessary. Gastric lavage may be needed if emesis does not occur, or if the child is unconscious. The exceptions to the rule of emesis are: (1) caustics, such as bleach or acids, which may be presumed from burning around the mouth if there is no adequate history; and (2) hydrocarbons such as turpentine and paraffin. In the case of caustics, the danger of gastric perforation is increased by emesis or lavage; hydrocarbons do little harm in the gastrointestinal tract, but inhalation of vomit may seriously damage the lungs.

Absorption may be discouraged by diluting the poison (milk is good and usually available), by giving an absorbent agent such as activated charcoal or by giving a specific antidote (e.g. desferrioxamine in iron poisoning). Excretion may be encouraged by the use of purgatives or forced diuresis in selected cases.

It is usually advisable to admit poisoned children to hospital for observation for at least a few hours. The Regional Poisons Information Centres provide helpful information and advice. (Their telephone numbers are listed in the British National Formulary.)

Drug abuse

The age at which youngsters become addicted to drugs continues to decrease. Alcohol and tobacco are the most frequently used though marijuana (cannabis) is not rare. *Solvent abuse*, in which substances such as glue, dry cleaning fluid and paints are inhaled, tends to cause similar effects to alcohol though there may be more marked visual and perceptual disturbances, as well as local lesions (sore and infected skin) around the nose and mouth as a result of a plastic bag or container being pressed to the face during inhalation. It is commonest in boys aged 13–15 years.

Chronic lead poisoning

Lead poisoning is uncommon in Britain. Lead water pipes have been largely replaced by copper, and drinking water is drawn from main supplies rather than storage tanks. Modern paints for interior decoration contain very little lead, and the British climate does not bring to mind the thought of peeling paint on the railings of a sun-baked verandah. Nevertheless, some risks still exist. Amateurs may use lead paints for home decorating or painting cots; lead dust may lie in the vicinity of smelting works or come home on the clothes of lead workers; and disused car batteries are a cheap, if dangerous, form of domestic fuel. Lead may be absorbed by ingestion, inhalation, or through the skin. There may be a history of ingestion of paint or dirt—*pica* (pica is the Latin name for magpie, a bird notorious for stealing and consuming almost anything).

Poisoning is usually chronic and the onset of symptoms is insidious. Early symptoms include abdominal colic, pallor, anaemia, irritability, anorexia and disturbed sleep. Later symptoms are predominantly neurological, including encephalopathy, neuropathy and seizures. Permanent brain damage may result in mental handicap and behavioural disorder. If the onset is more acute, encephalopathic features tend to predominate.

There is continuing debate and controversy about the significance of marginally elevated blood lead levels and their relationship to abnormal childhood behaviour.

CHILD ABUSE AND NEGLECT

Abuse: deliberately inflicted injury.

Neglect: inadequate or negligent parenting, failing to protect the child.

Many children suffer a combination of abuse and neglect. The definitions suggest that abuse is an active process and neglect a passive one but for most forms of abuse the parents, who are the usual perpetrators, contribute to the abuse by both active and passive roles. Thus the spouse who fails to intervene when their partner sexually abuses the child is a passive partner to the abuse and colluding with it. A parent who passively fails to provide food or love may also indulge in active physical assault.

A child is considered to be abused if he or she is treated by an adult in a way that is unacceptable in a given culture at a given time. It is important to recognize that children are treated differently not only in different countries but in different subcultures of one city and that there will be various opinions about what constitutes abuse. With the passage of time standards change: corporal punishment is less acceptable than it was 10 years ago. These factors contribute to the difficulties of defining child abuse and determining changes in its prevalence.

Types of abuse
1   Physical abuse (non-accidental injury).
2   Neglect.
3   Sexual abuse.
4   Emotional abuse.

Physical abuse
Such abuse is usually short-term and violent though it may be repetitive. Soft tissue injuries to the skin, ears and eyes are common as well as injuries to the joints and bones. The most common forms of injury are shown in Fig. 22.2. These are:

1   Bruising, especially of the face and trunk. The bruises may be multiple and of different ages. (But remember that a normal active toddler is likely to have five or six bruises of different ages on him, usually on the shins.)
2   Fractures, especially of the ribs, humerus and femur. Fractures at different stages of healing, denoting repetitive injury, or involving an infant are particularly suspicious.
3   Head injury, skull fracture and subdural haematoma may occur together or separately. Depressed and complicated (as opposed to simple linear) fractures are particularly suspicious. Retinal and subhyaloid haemorrhages may occur. The most severe head injuries will cause intraventricular and intracerebral haemorrhage leading to death or permanent brain damage.
4   Burns, either from cigarettes or holding a child close to a fire. Scalds, from immersion in very hot water (usually involving a hand, foot or buttock).

Helpful diagnostic features
These include:
1   Delay in seeking medical advice, or not seeking it at all.
2   The explanation of the accident is incompatible with the injury observed (a baby's skull does not fracture if he rolls off the sofa onto a carpeted floor).
3   The story of the accident varies between different informants.

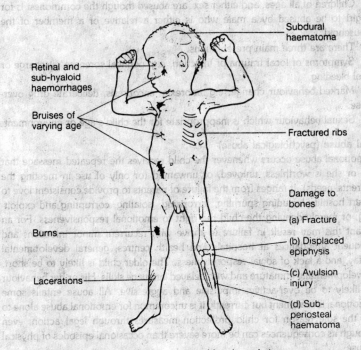

Fig. 22.2. Characteristic injuries caused by physical abuse.

4   The child is brought to the doctor by someone other than the person in whose presence the injury occurred.
5   Unusual parental behaviour with the parents being more interested in their own feelings, and in returning home, than in concern for the child. (Sometimes the parents will leave the child in hospital before the senior doctor has arrived.)
6   Abnormal parent–child interaction with the child looking frightened or withdrawn.

Neglect

Failing to provide the love, care, food or physical circumstances that will allow the child to grow and develop normally, or exposing a child to any kind of danger constitutes neglect.

Neglect and injury are closely associated and both are indications of parental inadequacy. The child may show evidence of poor standards of hygiene or nutrition; height and weight, when plotted on a growth record, may be well below the expected centile. Neglect is often combined with emotional abuse.

Sexual abuse

Child sexual abuse includes any use of children for the sexual gratification of adults. It ranges from inappropriate fondling and masturbation to intercourse and buggery. Children may be forced to appear in pornographic photographs or videos, or participate in sex rings or ritual abuse.

Children of all ages, and either sex, are abused though the commonest is for a girl to be abused by a male who is either a relative or a member of the household.

There are three main presentations:

1 Symptoms of local trauma or infection, e.g. perineal soreness, discharge or anal bleeding.

2 Marked behaviour change, e.g. anorexia, encopresis, deliberate drug over-dose.

3 Sexual behaviour which is inappropriate for the child's age or environment.

Emotional abuse (psychological abuse)

Emotional abuse occurs whenever the child receives the repeated message that he or she is worthless, unloved, or unwanted (or only of use in meeting the parents' needs). It ranges from the failure of parents to provide consistent love to overt hostility including spurning, terrorizing, isolating, corrupting and exploit-ing, or merely denying the child the right to emotional responsiveness. For an infant this may result in failure to thrive with recurrent minor infections and frequent attendances at hospitals and health centres, general developmental delay, and a lack of social responsiveness. The older child is likely to be short, developmentally immature and with delayed language skills. His or her behaviour is likely to be over-active, impulsive and aggressive. All abuse entails some emotional ill-treatment but currently it is uncommon for emotional abuse alone to be the sole reason for child protection measures through legal action, even though its consequences can be more severe than occasional episodes of physical abuse.

Munchausen syndrome by proxy

This term encompasses a range of behaviour, uusally by mothers, in which false illness is invented (for the child) for personal gain. It commonly includes both physical and emotional abuse. The spectrum extends from the anxious parent who perceives symptoms and signs that others do not observe; to 'doctor shopping' in which the mother seeks needless help from a succession of different doctors causing the child to have repetitive investigations and treatments; 'enforced invalidism' in which parents who have a genuinely ill or disabled child increase the degree of disability to ensure the child is incapacitated and does not participate in normal schooling and activities, to the extreme end of the spectrum of 'fabricated illness' in which the parent not only invents a false illness story but fabricates physical signs, alters health records and, at times, poisons or suffocates the child. The consequences for the child in terms of unpleasant and harmful investigations and treatments, the induction of genuine disease, and the effects of poisoning or suffocation can be disastrous. Furthermore, the child may be encouraged to be a chronic invalid and believe himself or herself to be disabled and unable to attend school and may develop somatoform behaviour (e.g. Munchausen syndrome) as as adult.

Prevalence

Four per cent of children up to the age of 12 are notified to social service departments because of suspected abuse. Some of that abuse may be mild but at least 1 child per 1000 under the age of 4 suffers severe physical abuse, e.g. fractures, brain haemorrhage or mutilation. This week at least 4 children in Britain will die as a result of abuse or neglect.

There is some evidence that there may have been an increase in child abuse in the past 5 years but the apparent increase may be more the result of greater unwillingness by society to tolerate child abuse, increased public awareness and professional recognition.

Perpetrators

Parents are the usual abusers. Physical abuse, emotional abuse and neglect are often inflicted by both parents. Sex abuse is more common by men, and poisoning, suffocation and Munchausen syndrome by proxy by the mother.

Abuse occurs in all sections of society. It is recognized more readily in poor families and probably occurs more commonly in those families—'Destructiveness is the outcome of unlived life.' It is more common if the parents themselves were abused as children and, particularly, if they lacked love and respect from their own parents.

The motives for abuse are complex. We can all understand how a weary parent in an overcrowded home, where the children are on top of one another, and the father is on shift work attempting to sleep, hits out impatiently at a fractious overdemanding child. However, much abuse is repetitive and, seemingly, premeditated. Often it is an expression of the parent's inner violence and their wish to exert power over their child. It is common for normal parents to have mixed feelings about their children and to have moments when they hate their child. Most parents can control their feelings but a minority injure their child during those feelings of hatred. They are not suffering mental illness but they do have a personality disorder.

Management

All doctors should have a low threshold for suspecting abuse and be prepared to refer the child for more detailed assessment. A careful record should be kept of the initial consultation including the history, and who provided it, and drawings of any injuries. Subsequently, photographs may be taken or a skeletal X-ray survey performed to detect unsuspected fractures. A telephone call to the duty social worker for the district will reveal whether or not the child is already on the Child Protection Register and considered 'at risk' for abuse. That would make the likelihood of abuse greater.

If abuse is likely the doctor (or other concerned person) will contact the Social Services Department who usually convene a *case conference* (Fig. 22.3). All professional workers who know the family are invited including the GP, health visitor and school teacher. The aim is to form a clear picture of the child and family relationships and then, making the child's interests paramount, recommendations are made for the child's future safety, including decisions about future legal proceedings. If the child is in imminent danger an *Emergency Protection Order* (formerly a *Place of Safety Order*) may be sought from a magistrate. This allows the child to be detained in a hospital or foster home whilst enquiries are made.

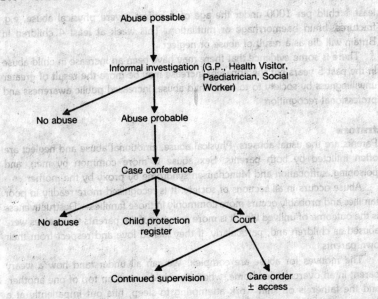

Fig. 22.3. The usual course of investigation of an allegation of abuse. The original allegation might be made by relatives of the child, neighbours, the GP or health visitor, hospital staff, police, education or social services. The more formal investigation commences with the multidisciplinary case conference.

Subsequent court action may be needed to take a child into the care of the local authority if the risk of further abuse at home is too great (see p. 9). More commonly the child is placed on the Child Protection Register and skilled help arranged for the families so that the child can be supervised at home and the family helped to modify their behaviour. This help and supervision is normally provided by local authority social workers or the National Society for the Prevention of Cruelty to Children (NSPCC). Further abuse occurs in up to 20% of cases; the recurrence rate is a sensitive index of the effectiveness of management.

The police are represented at case conferences and may be asked to investigate more serious or difficult cases. However, a minority of cases end with a criminal prosecution. When that does happen, guilty mothers are usually given a suspended sentence or made the subject of a probation order whereas guilty fathers usually receive a custodial sentence; it is an interesting reflection of how society currently views the problem of child abuse.

SUDDEN INFANT DEATH SYNDROME (SIDS, COT DEATH)

The sudden death of an infant which is unexpected by history, and in which thorough post-mortem examination fails to demonstrate an adequate cause, occurs in 2 per 1000 live births. In the UK, cot death constitutes about one-fifth of infant deaths, and is the commonest category after the age of 1 month.

Most occur at home between the ages of 4 weeks and 4 months, in urban rather than rural areas, during the night, and in late winter and early spring, when community respiratory infections are most prevalent. They are frequently preceded by symptoms of minor illness; they are more common in males, in twins, in infants of low birthweight, and in the socially and economically deprived. The infants' mothers tend to be younger and to have had more children when compared with controls.

SIDS is a categorization rather than an explanation. It is a non-diagnosis, the label being applied when no reason for death can be found—even after autopsy. A hundred years ago it was customary to attribute most cot deaths to 'overlaying' (suffocation) by the mother, whether accidental or deliberate. A small proportion of SIDS deaths today are caused by parents but it is likely to be well under 10%—the great majority of parents are in no way to blame. Many hypotheses have been proposed to explain SIDS: it is likely that several different causes will be identified eventually. Popular theories include abnormalities of the cardiac and ventilatory control systems. It is postulated that a lethal combination of intrinsic and extrinsic factors arises at a time when the infant is passing through a stage of increased physiological vulnerability. Possible extrinsic factors include overheating and sleeping in the prone position.

Sudden unexpected death causes a profound family crisis and the bereaved parents needs expert counselling and help. Commonly such parents are lent an apnoea alarm when they have a subsequent baby; though this may be reassuring, evidence is lacking that the alarms prevent cot death.

FURTHER READING

Golding J, Limerick S and MacFarlane A. *Sudden Infant Death*. Open Books.
Jackson RH. *Children, The Environment and Accidents*. Pitman Medical.
Jones DN. *Understanding Child Abuse*. Hodder and Stoughton.
Meadow R. *ABC of Child Abuse*. BMA Publications.
Porter R. *Child Sexual Abuse within the Family*. Ciba Foundation.

Appendices

1 MEASUREMENT AND CONVERSION

To Metric

One ounce	= 28.4 grams (g)
One pound	= 0.45 kilogram (kg)
One fluid ounce	= 28.4 millilitres (ml)
One pint	= 0.56 litre (l)*
One inch	= 2.54 centimetres (cm)

From Metric

One kilogram	= 2.2 pounds (lb)
One litre	= 1.76 pints
One centimetre	= 0.39 inch (in)

2 FURTHER READING

At the end of most chapters we have listed books for further reading or reference. In addition there are many comprehensive paediatric textbooks and specialist monographs—more than enough to suit all tastes. Those that we find particularly useful and which are likely to be in the local library are given below.

Large comprehensive textbooks

Behrman RE and Vaughan. *Nelson's Textbook of Paediatrics*. WB Saunders.
Forfar JO and Arneil GC. *Textbook of Paediatrics*. Churchill Livingstone.

Other books

Godfrey S and Baum JD. *Clinical Paediatric Physiology*. Blackwell Scientific Publications.
Henley A. *Asian Patients in Hospital and at Home*. Kings Fund Publishing Office, London.
Mitchell RG. *Child health in the Community*. Churchill Livingstone.
Nixon HH and O'Donnell B. *The Essentials of Paediatric Surgery*. Heinemann.
Rutter M and Hersov L. *Child and Adolescent Psychiatry*. Blackwell Scientific Publications.
Smith DW. *Recognizable Patterns of Human Malformation*. WB Saunders.
Clinics in Developmental Medicine—a series of monographs on neurological and developmental aspects of children. MacKeith Press.

Reviews

Topical reviews on selected subjects are available in the following periodic publications.

---

* The USA pint contains 16 fluid ounces, i.e. 0.45 litre.

Recent Advances in Paediatrics. Churchill Livingstone.
The Pediatric Clinics of North America. WB Saunders.

Books for parents

Illingworth C and Illingworth R. *Babies and Young Children*. Churchill Livingstone.
Jolly H. *The Book of Child Care*. Allen and Unwin.
Spock B. *Dr Spock's Baby and Child Care*. W.H.Allen.

Index

Page numbers in *italic* type refer to figures

251